Looking for the Golden Thread

Enriching the practice of T'ai Chi Ch'üan through lineage, experience, and reflection

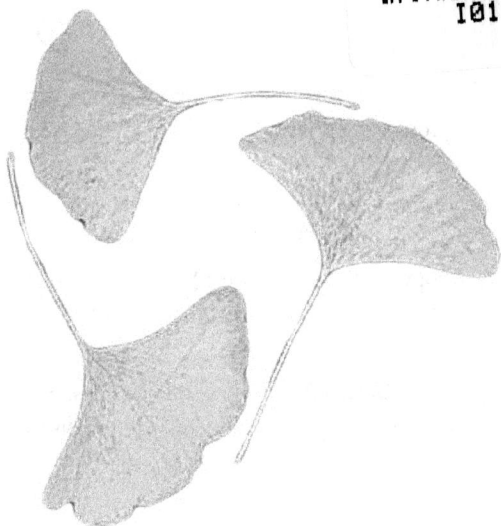

Faith Burton Gregor

Publisher: Northern Star TC, LLC
Editor: Linda Wolf, Network Publishing Partners, Inc.
Publishing Consultant and Cover Designer:
Sedrik Newbern, Newbern Consulting, LLC
Author Photo: Aurora Walker

Printed in the United States of America
First Edition: July 2024

Author's Note:
In several of the "Narrative/Lived Experience" sections, names have been
changed to protect the privacy of the individuals referenced therein.

From *The Essence and Applications of Taijiquan* by Yang Chengfu, translated
by Louis Swaim, published by Blue Snake Books, an imprint of North
Atlantic Books, copyright © 2005 Louis Swaim. Reprinted by permission of
Blue Snake Books c/o North Atlantic Books.

From *Looking for The Golden Needle* by Gerda Geddes, published by Manna-
Media, an imprint of Mannamead Press, copyright ©1991 Gerda Geddes. Reprinted by permission of Harriet Devlin.

From *Tai Chi Chuan Classical Yang Style: The Complete Form and Qigong* by
Yang, Jwing-Ming. published by YMAA Publication Center, copyright © 1999
Yang, Jwing-Ming. Reprinted by permission of YMAA Publication Center.

ISBN Paperback: 979-8-9908646-0-3
Library of Congress Control Number: 2024911972

For my teachers, students,
and companions in the t'ai chi ch'üan community,
with love and gratitude

Contents

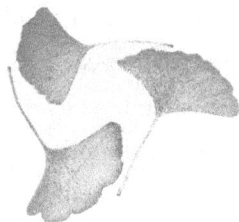

Introduction

In January 1999, I attended my first lesson in t'ai chi ch'üan. On a frigid winter evening, I met my wonderful teacher (and current teaching partner), Maedée Duprès. She started out by asking each attendee how they became interested in the practice. For me, it felt like t'ai chi ch'üan had invited me – offering a gentle yet compelling suggestion to move through the world in a different way.

Throughout the following year, as we slowly learned the form, Ms. Duprès often referred to her own teacher, Gerda Geddes. Ms. Geddes was internationally renowned as the first Caucasian woman to teach t'ai chi ch'üan in Europe. We came to know Ms. Geddes's work through her book *Looking for The Golden Needle*.

While we learned the movements and sequences of the t'ai chi ch'üan, Ms. Duprès deftly wove passages and concepts from *Looking for The Golden Needle* into our lessons on the sequences and movements of t'ai chi ch'üan. This resulted in a wonderful experience of mind-body learning. When I started teaching t'ai chi ch'üan myself in 2008, I hoped to pass that experience forward by honoring the lineage of the Yang style t'ai chi ch'üan and the wonderful teachers in my life.

In *Looking for The Golden Needle*, Ms. Geddes portrays t'ai chi ch'üan as an allegorical journey. She interprets the flowing movements of the form as a metaphorical and symbolic enactment of birth, childhood, adult life, later years, and at the end of life, release and freedom. She also relates her own experience of encountering t'ai chi ch'üan in China in the 1940s, and then later learning it from a student of Yang Chengfu, the grandson of the founder of Yang style t'ai chi ch'üan.

Geddes's book has been invaluable to me throughout my decades of t'ai chi practice. It's also a powerful narrative of living one's life in balance and harmony. *Looking for the Golden Thread* was inspired by *Looking for The Golden Needle*. Simply stated, my intent is to connect readers to the joy of t'ai chi ch'üan. That joy encompasses physical, mental, and spiritual well-being for long-time practitioners, beginners, and anyone who would like to know more about this ancient martial art.

Looking for the Golden Thread is a guide to support a journey of body, mind, and spirit through the practice of t'ai chi ch'üan. I like to think of it as being useful in the same way a book identifying flowers or birds would be when tucked into a daypack before setting out for a hike. It is not a complete and detailed work of instruction. For that, I would advise prospective students to find a qualified teacher in an in-person setting.

Each chapter covers one sequence selected from the three-part, 108-movement Yang style. Each includes three sections discussing aspects of that sequence: symbolism, tradition, and background; narrative/lived experience; and reflections of mind, body, and intent. These 13 selected sequences offer a taste of the 108-movement form and invite further exploration in a class or group.

Each chapter also contains a still photo from the featured sequence, a photo to suggest the relationship of nature to the practice of t'ai chi ch'üan, and a "moving illustration" video of that sequence.

My intent is to shine a light on the traditions and the extraordinary teachers of my lineage, share insights and stories from my own experiences and those of my students, and explore reflections on how the practice might enhance our whole selves.

In my experience as a teacher and a student, it has been my delight to witness this centuries-old practice of t'ai chi ch'üan sparkling with life in the present moment – while discovering the rich tradition and symbolism, inviting it to seep into life experiences, and appreciating the quiet, powerful energy and joy of each movement.

It has also been inspiring to find my own place within the metaphorical journey...and even more inspiring to hear about the experiences of others. I'm grateful to all who shared their stories and I offer this book as a loving tribute to students, teachers, lineage, and tradition. They have all changed my life in ways I never imagined.

ABOUT THE VIDEOS

The QR code links you to 13 videos. Each one corresponds to the the 13 chapters of *Looking for the Golden Thread*.

These videos are provided for illustrative purposes only and are not intended to be instructional or a substitute for professional medical advice, diagnosis, or treatment. The content is not designed to teach t'ai chi ch'üan or any other form of exercise. Always seek the advice of your physician or other qualified health provider with any questions you may have regarding a medical condition or exercise program. Never disregard professional medical advice or delay in seeking it because of something you have seen in these videos. If you wish to learn t'ai chi ch'üan, we strongly recommend seeking in-person instruction from a qualified teacher. The creators of these videos assume no responsibility for injuries or damages resulting from the use or misuse of the information provided.

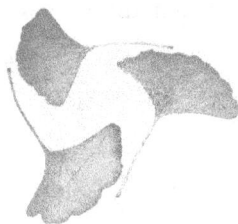

Chapter 1

Grasping the Bird's Tail

Symbolism, Tradition, and Background

T'ai chi ch'üan is full of bird symbols and metaphors. We can reflect on the beauty of bird movements and emulate them in our practice. We can also evoke the names as cues to help us remember the movements and keep track of their order.

In the very first movement, Grasping the Bird's Tail, all these elements come into play.

Think about the physical characteristics, nature, and appearance of an actual bird's tail. It is nimble, strong, and supple, with each feather separate and distinct, yet all acting as a unit to balance, support, and steer the bird. We bring our attention to our hand and think about how it might illustrate and "perform" the shape and function of the bird's tail as described above. From the supple wrist, the fingers actively extend downward. There is a little space between each one. This allows air currents to flow through and suggests a bird's tail – an organized group of feathers with a purpose, but not rigidly held.

We can also link the shape to the intent. This is an important principle for all movements, and it's interesting to learn how different practitioners go about this, essentially "setting the stage" for the mind, body, and spirit to participate in each movement.

Dr. Yang, Jwing-Ming is a renowned t'ai chi master and the author of *Tai Chi Chuan Classical Yang Style.* He often describes and teaches the movements from the standpoint of offensive and defensive strategies with an opponent. Here is an excerpt from his narrative on Grasp the Sparrow's Tail.

> Grasp sparrow's tail in Chinese is "lan que wei." "Lan" means grasp or seize. This implies that when you apply this technique you not only intercept your opponent's strike, but also grasp him. A sparrow's tail is very light and fragile, and also sensitive and mobile. Therefore, when you grasp the sparrow's tail you must be cautious and sensitive, and you cannot use muscular strength. (Dr. Yang, Jwing-Ming, 1999, page 194)[1]

For another viewpoint on bringing intent to movement, consider this description written by Gerda Geddes in *Looking for The Golden Needle.*

> In the opening sequences of the T'ai chi Ch'üan, as we leave the firmly rooted standing position, we step out into a movement called **Grasping the Bird's Tail.** The bird is thought of as the messenger between Heaven and Earth and this grasping of the bird's tail indicates the individual's first awareness and curiosity for his wider surroundings. The bird also symbolizes air and spirit, so it seems that as we become more conscious we feel ourselves as moving through air, being illumined by spirit.[2]

Narrative/Lived Experience

In December 2007, my father and I took a three-day trip to Bosque del Apache National Wildlife Refuge to see more than 40,000 snow geese and 10,000 greater sandhill cranes at their annual winter home. Bosque del Apache is a fairly remote spot near Socorro, New Mexico, about 80 miles south of Albuquerque. The refuge surrounds a wide, flat, and open area on the Rio Grande River floodplain. After centuries of flood-control measures had altered the river's natural rhythm, it was restored in the 1930s as a wildlife habitat by the Civilian Conservation Corps. As the refuge website notes:

> Situated between the Chupadera Mountains to the west and the San Pascual Mountains to the east, the 57,331 acre Bosque del Apache was established in 1939 to provide a critical stopover site for migrating waterfowl. The refuge is well known for the tens of thousands of cranes, geese, and ducks who winter here each year. Over 30,000 acres of Bosque del Apache are designated wilderness. ... Today, our staff manages water to create wetlands like when the river ran wild. These seasonal wetlands re-create the types of habitats that both year-round and migratory wildlife need to thrive. Using gates and ditches, water is moved from the river through fields, marshes, and ponds, and then back to the river to mimic natural flooding cycles.[3]

The refuge administration manages soil, native trees, and plants to support the habitat. Local farmers and refuge staff grow corn, millet, winter wheat, clover, and native plants on the refuge for the wintering cranes and geese, as well as for hundreds of other migratory and local bird species.

Mid-November to early February is the peak time for migrating and wintering waterfowl. Visitors come to lookout points on the refuge at sunrise or sunset, when the flocks of cranes and geese that roost in the refuge "commute" to or from the local fields where they feed.

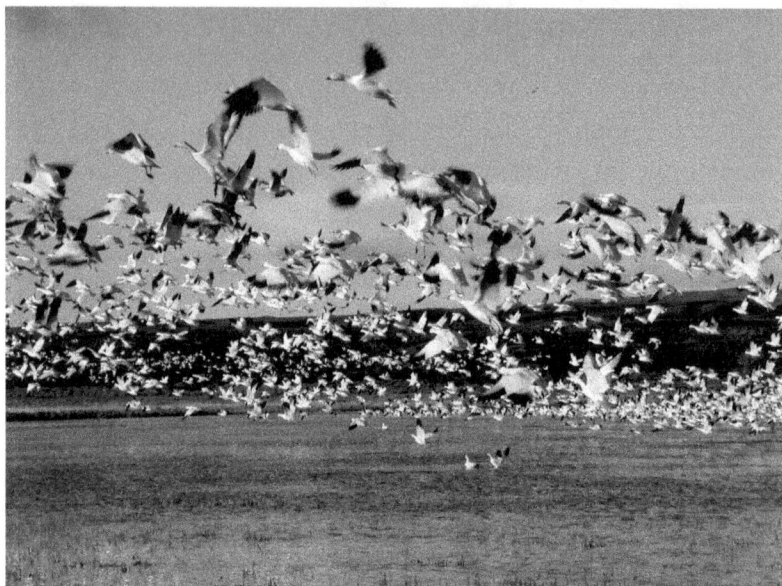

Snow geese at Bosque Del Apache National Wildlife Refuge

I was looking forward to finally getting to see this spectacular natural event as described to me by my father, who had witnessed it several times. His routine was to pack up his Suzuki Samurai, leave Denver around 5 a.m., drive the 500-plus miles to the refuge in time for the birds' evening flight, sleep overnight at a local bed and breakfast, watch the morning flight, and immediately afterward, drive straight back to Denver. That added up to 16 hours of driving time, seven hours of sleep, and two hours of bird-watching.

From my standpoint, that ratio needed a little adjustment to be comfortable. As a combination birthday and Christmas treat for us both, I arranged for two nights' accommodation, airfare, and a rental car in Albuquerque. We even scored a bulkhead seat for the hour-long flight.

That afternoon we settled in at our bed and breakfast, then drove to the nearby refuge. The area was peaceful and empty. The flat, sparse, and spacious landscape softened and faded to the horizon in the lingering mist and clouds from an earlier rain shower. A few dozen sandhill cranes strolled around on the damp dirt road and in the rushes bordering the river and lagoons. We drove to the lookout, one of several along the few roads through the sanctuary. My father looked expectantly to the west.

Then out of the emptiness came a sound I'd never heard before, faint at first and then gradually flooding our auditory landscape. It was a powerful upwelling of sound, emerging from a place in the sky just beyond the horizon and growing nearer, clearer, and louder.

I was hearing the calls of the snow geese on their evening flight, arriving from the nearby millet and alfalfa fields to the lakes and ponds where they'd spend the night protected from predators. We stood transfixed, our ears and bodies absorbing the deep roar of a 10,000-member avian orchestra.

At that point, the sky became thickly stippled with moving dots. The dots grew larger and transformed into dense crowds of white snow geese. Their destination was a lagoon behind us, but a few of them landed on the water in front of our observation point.

Watching a waterbird land, whether it's a goose, crane, or duck, is pure wonder. Once the bird has chosen its landing point, it slows, descends, changes from flight posture to landing posture, makes contact feet first, and folds its wings. This all happens as smoothly and gracefully as a ballet dancer gliding across a stage.

Most waterfowl have short, stout tails with feathers that can fan out widely. Their tails are adapted to each bird's individual feeding habits, and for those that dive to forage, their tails can also act as rudders under the water. But it is in the air that the subtle, strong, precise steering and balancing work done by the tail are most wonderfully apparent to human admirers.

Photos I took that afternoon show more of the amazing traits of tails. In one image, sandhill cranes are cruising in for a landing on the lagoon in the late-afternoon twilight. Their grey bodies are a little paler than the background of bushes and the rapidly dimming winter sky. Their outstretched necks in front, and their straight legs behind, are graceful and aerodynamic. Their bodies and short tails form a neat almond shape in between. The tails finish out the back end of the almond's gentle transition from wide to narrow. The whole unit undulates gently with each flap of the wing to help deliver the tremendous energy needed to fly.

The next morning at 5 a.m., we drove in subzero darkness to the overlook, warming our hands with a thermos of coffee as we waited for the cranes to lift off for the day. They did so in groups of ten or so, like silent, shimmering ghosts. Their slim grey bodies rose from the water, framed by the morning sky and winter vegetation turning reddish-gold with the sunrise.

At a nearby lagoon, the snow geese were preparing for another stunning performance. Hundreds of them were closely gathered in stillness on the surface of the water. Then, one black-tipped pair of snowy wings fanned the air. About a minute later, they were all airborne.

My photo of the lift-off shows hundreds of birds, moving together but each in its own sequence of flight. It was a thrilling experience to watch them as a whole community of movement – wings stirring the air, bodies moving forward in the collective energy of flying. As with the cranes, tails and wings acted as a unit, bending to create a downdraft, lifting to bring buoyancy of body and spirit into the crisp, blue, early winter sky.

Reflections of Mind, Body, and Intent

At the Bosque del Apache Annual Crane Festival, I saw and felt pure, serene beauty, energy, and power. I might never get to experience that again, but I was lucky enough to get a few pictures. Like all photos, they captured the moment but not the majesty. That sense of awe lives in my memory, still present but only a faint echo of the real event.

Performing the sequence of Grasping the Bird's Tail, my hands draw apart, evoking the memory of the birds' magic interaction of muscle, energy, and air. The hands tell the story. They also connect with each other's energy in passing. The lifting hand, with fingers trailing, becomes the bird in flight. Its yang energy rises to the heavens, while the

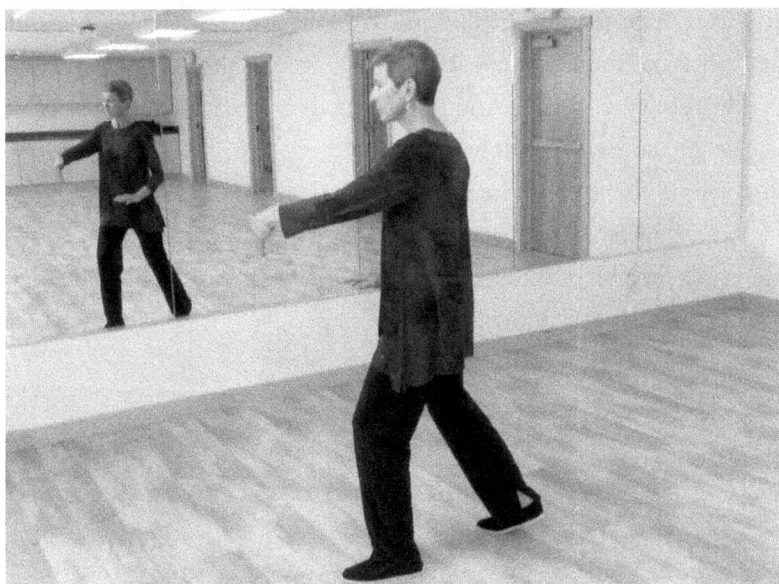

The fingers of the rising hand evoke the feathers of a bird's tail.

sinking yin hand returns to the earth. Then, yin and yang return to their primordial relationship as the two arcs of the circle. Resting, rising, or sinking, the space between the two hands is the supple, powerful essence of life.

This movement feels buoyant, agile, and strong, and it suggests a child's seeking, adventurous intent. The eighth of Yang Chengfu's Ten Points, "Inside and outside coordinate," speaks to this sense of lightness. "If you can raise the spirit, then the movements will be naturally agile." [4]

The smooth shifts of weight and direction in Grasping the Bird's Tail invite the body into a sense of unity. To further encourage that unity and harmony, imagine a string of pearls suspending your head from above. The head rests easily on the spine, each vertebra a glossy pearl. The neck is long and supple. The upper and lower ends of the spine gently lengthen away from each other, with space between each vertebra to support easy rotation. Simply intend for that space to be there, regardless of the variations brought on by age and circumstances.

Visualize openness in the spine and in all the joints, where body, mind, and spirit collaborate to create fluid, strong, and flexible movement.

In the same manner, use the intent to create width in the hip so the weight softly pours down into your feet. The whole leg is a strong and supple channel for the unbroken flow of chi.

The fingers are soft and curved, with just a little space between them. Then, a breeze could dance with the feathers of the bird's tail to encourage agility, stability, and buoyancy.

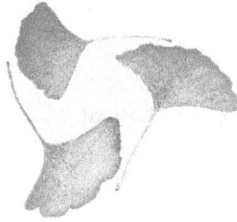

Chapter 2

Bird's Beak/Single Whip

Symbolism, Tradition, and Background

This sequence makes its first appearance early in the form and is repeated nine more times. These repetitions offer many opportunities to polish the movements of Bird's Beak and Single Whip, and to reflect on the meaning.

Throughout her book *Looking for The Golden Needle,* Gerda Geddes evokes joy, profundity, and wonder in her description of the movements of the t'ai chi ch'üan. For example, here is her word portrait of Single Whip.

The last gesture of each of the eleven sequences is called *The Single Whip* where one arm makes the movement of a whip, the fingers of the other close together to portray a bird's beak. As each of these sequences is complete in itself, it would be appropriate here to quote Chuang Tzu:

The bird opens its beak and sings its note,
Then the beak comes together again in silence;
So nature and the living meet together in stillness,
Like the closing of the bird's beak after its song.[1]

The words are a window into the harmony, natural balance, and serenity of the Taoist worldview. It's as if the mind is taking a leisurely stroll through a gallery of Chinese landscape paintings, one beautiful image flowing into the next. The memory of such a visit might then seep into one's t'ai chi practice, inviting the body to move with gentle flow and appreciate each sequence in its turn.

Geddes's description of the Single Whip evokes an important element in t'ai chi practice that is present in many styles and lineages.

The symbol relates to the felt presence of energy between the two hands. My teacher Maedée Duprès sometimes leads students in an exercise that warms the hands, adds agility, and demonstrates that presence, or chi. (In this book I've chosen to use the simplified transcription of this Chinese word, but other sources spell it as qi. Both are widely used.)

Chi is defined as "vital energy that is held to animate the body internally and is of central importance in some Eastern systems of medical treatment (such as acupuncture) and of exercise or self-defense (such as tai chi)."[2]

To discover the flow of chi, sit or stand comfortably. Close your eyes and rub your hands together, gently but briskly, for about ten seconds. Next, with the palms facing each other, about two inches apart and with relaxed fingers pointing away from you, slowly draw the hands apart. Notice the energy "current" between the two hands. Part of that is the radiant physical warmth you've generated, but as the hands get more distant, the warmth dissipates but the energy current remains.

This hand exercise is a simple way to experience the presence of chi. It's like show-and-tell for the mind. As the mind experiences the body's movement, it experiences the physical manifestation of chi. This gives the mind a tangible connection with chi and a bridge to it through a lived experience. This simple and relaxing activity establishes and strengthens that connecting bridge, so that we become more familiar with chi and how it moves and works.

With Geddes's description of the Single Whip gesture and the words of Chuang Tzu, we might then visualize our hands drawing out a "golden thread": a powerful and intentional energy connection to enrich the sequence with grace, flow, intent, patience and restraint. The thread is slowly drawn out, but not broken by pulling too hard.

The golden thread visualization addresses another important element in all styles of t'ai chi: the energy and movement of the two hands in relationship with each other. As with other common elements, this is expressed in various ways among the styles, lineages, and individual teachers.

Yang Chengfu, grandson of Yang Luchan, founded the Yang style as it is widely taught today. He was my teacher's teacher's teacher's teacher – my t'ai chi great-great-grandfather, one might say. His 1934 book, *The Essence and Applications of Taijiquan*, contains many references to the connective powers of energy, thread, silk – and hands.

In a section titled "The Mental Elucidation of the Thirteen Postures," he writes:

Leading the movements to and fro, the *qi* adheres to the back, then collects into the spine. Within, consolidate the spirit of vitality. Without, express tranquillity and ease. Step like a cat walking. Mobilize energy *(jin)* as though drawing silk.[3]

His description of Single Whip touches on the idea of hands in relationship.

...collect the five fingers of the right hand, dropping them down and making a hook hand. At this moment, the left palm stops for an instant before the waist, forming an embrace with the hook hand, the heart of the palm facing upward.[4]

The chiefly oral traditions of t'ai chi are slowly making their way into written records and descriptions. This is an ongoing and often inconsistent process. To help myself out during decades of learning and honing the form, I've often used symbols and metaphors that put my mind and intent in a happy place. This fosters the relaxation and openness which are so supportive to my practice.

With that in mind, "drawing out a golden thread" is similar to what other styles refer to as "spinning" or "reeling" silk. Here is an insight from the Yang Family Tai Chi Discussion Board.

...in the Yang style what we have is twisting and continuous motion. It has the chan ssu jing element [from Chen style tai chi], but we do not call it "chan ssu jing"... Whether you call it "Silk Reeling," "Pulling Silk," "Open, rounded, and extended," or simply "Turn waist, rotate hips, rotate arms..." I believe there's a Shakespeare quote that is pertinent here: A rose, by any other name... so...There you go. Call it whatever you want to call it. Silk Reeling. Pulling Silk. Open, rounded, extended. Turning Waist. Rolling hips. Circling. Rotate arms. One family. One art. Have fun with whatever it is you call it.[5]

Narrative/Lived Experience

I am a Westerner whose mental, emotional, and spiritual landscapes have been influenced by a variety of worldviews. I practiced t'ai chi ch'üan for about six years before embarking on a year-long teacher certification program with five colleagues and my extraordinary instructor, Maedée Duprès, founder of Open Wings T'ai Chi Studio. Part of our curriculum was to research and present a topic. I chose an idea dear to my heart: nature as a bridge to connect west to east in order to learn, absorb, and honor t'ai chi's beloved, centuries-old movements and traditions. For me, this was more than a research topic, it was – and is – a way of life. The presence of nature, and my place in the physical universe, have always been central to my learning and teaching. Here are a few examples.

Coaxing a Drop of Sweetness from the Honeysuckle Stem

The "golden thread" visual doesn't need to be a thread spun on a loom. As I prepared to teach a class on a hot and sunny June morning several years ago, the honeysuckle vine blooming in my back yard triggered a childhood memory. Growing up in a part of rural New Jersey

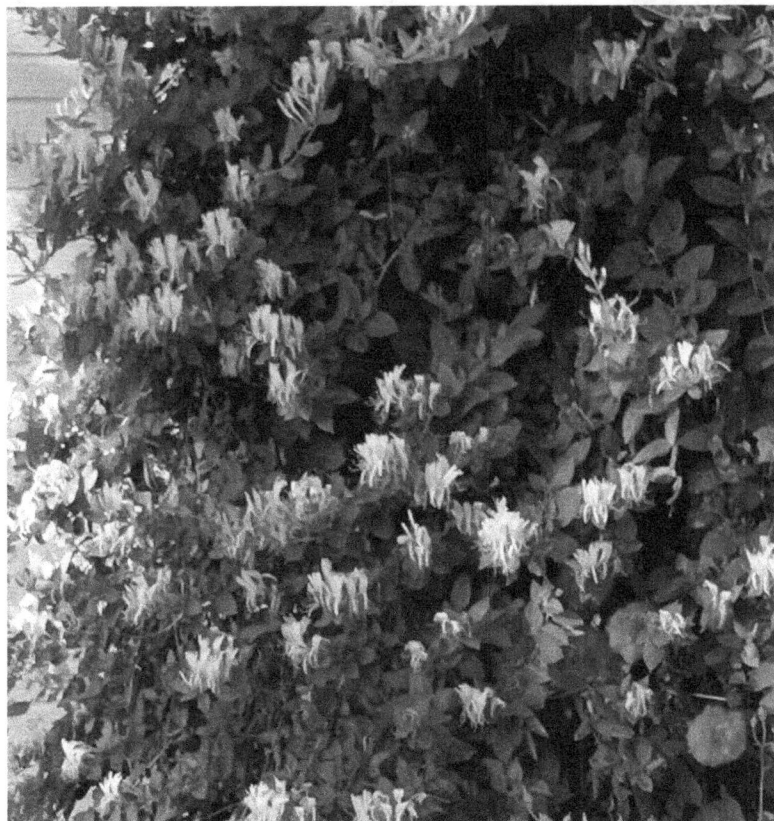

On this honeysuckle vine, each flower holds a tiny, delicious sip of nectar.

where honeysuckles are abundant, I learned how to sip nectar from the fragrant flowers. Here's how it works. First, pick a flower from the vine. Then hold the flower with one hand, and with the other hand, pinch just above the stem end so that you just break through the neck of the trumpet. Then, as you carefully pull the small end away from the rest of the flower, you'll see the central "string," or style. Keep pulling gently until a delicious drop appears. Then enjoy the nectar of the gods!

Floating on that pleasant memory, I connected with the t'ai chi idea of "drawing out the golden thread." I thought my students would enjoy a real-life example of what might seem like an ambiguous concept, so I snipped off a few honeysuckle flowers, took them to class and demonstrated the technique. I can't say whether the "drawing silk" metaphor migrated into their practice, but they all enjoyed their taste of nectar.

A Little Levity

As residents of the physical world, we are subject to its physical laws: momentum, gravity, and the rest. Examining how our bodies interact with the world can enhance our awareness of the connecting, spinning threads of energy. This doesn't have to be a painstaking, scientific endeavor. Patience and a sense of humor go a long way when it comes to grappling with the whys, wherefores, and limitations of our bodies and minds.

I like to figure out ways to get my students to laugh. That often happens without me trying. I am apt to get lost or mess up in front of a roomful of people, and in my early experiences as an instructor, I learned that teaching is a lot more fun if I don't take myself too seriously.

Teaching goofs are good for a laugh, as are unexpectedly silly metaphors. Here's one of my favorite stories I tell students, to illustrate movement in a relaxed and nimble manner.

There is a small, inexpensive wooden toy, usually a human or four-legged animal figure, that consists of hollow tubes of wood, connected through the cores with elastic string, held taut underneath. The figure stands at attention on a small wooden platform. Push up a wooden disc from beneath and the elastic releases, which causes the figure to collapse in a comical, exaggerated fashion. Release the disc and the elastic tightens, springing the figure back to rigid attention.

Once the visual is established, I ask students to imagine that they're holding one of those toys. Then I ask them to imagine that they've placed their fingers on the disc but haven't exerted any pressure…they're just in that moment of intent. That's how to be relaxed! Not held too tight – when the wooden figure is completely tense – and not too loose – when the figure collapses. At that point in the story, I demonstrate a tightly held body, then release my muscles and sink down to the floor.

Usually I see heads nodding as people relate to the imagery. That part is clear and familiar, and from that point we can examine the role of intent, which is very important but quite nuanced. When a t'ai chi practitioner gets a sense of how the intent directs movement, that's a big step…a taste of chi itself.

Patience, the Best Medicine

I now see chi in everyday American life, and I see how I unknowingly connected to some of its attributes long before I had ever heard of t'ai chi ch'üan.

When I was 12, I joined a 4-H sewing club. 4-H (Head, Heart, Hands and Health) is a youth organization affiliated with state universities. Its mission is to bring the universities' resources and services to rural communities. These clubs teach useful skills in a hands-on setting, such as raising sheep and cattle, gardening, and sewing.

I was fortunate to have a talented, creative, and patient club leader who was an accomplished seamstress and tailor. Thanks to her expert instruction, I learned this skill and sewed many of my own clothes in high school, my wedding dress, a sport coat for my husband, all sorts of Halloween outfits, costumes for high school and college theater productions, and several generations of curtains for the house I've lived in for decades. I had a great time sewing all those projects and saved thousands of dollars along the way.

There's an obvious physical connection between sewing with thread and "drawing out the golden thread." But another important aspect of successful sewing has something in common with t'ai chi: patience – particularly, the patience to learn when it's time to set the work aside for another day.

It took quite a while and quite a bit of frustration to figure out how to stop when tired. Usually I would grit my teeth and push on past the mistake to an arbitrary stopping point, only to make more mistakes. Eventually there was no choice but rip out many seams, put the work away, brush off the setback, and start fresh.

In my early days of learning t'ai chi ch'üan, I often reached a point where my brain and body felt stuck, like a pinball machine on "tilt." The harder I tried to master a sequence, the more I ran up against a frustrating sense of frozen disconnection. In order to move forward, I had to stop, breathe, back up, and start again from the original point of deviation. Mistakes are inevitable, but we don't have to get swept up in the energy of frustration. So whether I'm sewing or practicing t'ai chi, I try to keep the thread comfortable and straight, keep the puckers to a minimum, and bring an abundant supply of patience.

The Power of Place and Weaving Connections

In my quest to connect the threads, there's another wonderful, simple method that never fails me. It's the notion that there is a power in "place." A beloved example for me is William Butler Yeats's poem "The Lake Isle of Innisfree." When I read this poem, or call it up in my memory, the threads of place gently gather me in and I am home – gently cradled in the images it evokes. Each line of the poem is like a silken thread to connect me to nature's sacred and powerful space.

The Lake Isle of Innisfree

I will arise and go now, and go to Innisfree,
And a small cabin build there, of clay and wattles made;
Nine bean-rows will I have there, a hive for the honey-bee,
And live alone in the bee-loud glade.
And I shall have some peace there, for peace comes dropping slow,
Dropping like the veils of the morning to where the cricket sings;
There midnight's all a-glimmer, and noon a purple glow,
And evening full of the linnet's wings.
I will arise and go now, for always, night and day,
I hear lake water lapping with low sounds by the shore;
While I stand on the roadway, or on the pavements gray,
I hear it in the deep heart's core.[6]

We can abide in a place of beauty and harmonious balance, whether it's on the Lake Isle of Innisfree in Ireland's Lough Gill, as Yeats writes about, or whether it's standing in a gallery and letting the mind wander through a mist-shrouded Chinese landscape painting. Stop and rest in the beauty ahead, behind, above, and below. There you may find that the ten directions of the t'ai chi can inform your practice and perhaps your worldview as well.

Reflections of Mind, Body, and Intent

Strings, threads, and connecting energy all travel a common path. In t'ai chi ch'üan, energy moves out on a path from the center of the body to the extremities, then returns to the center to renew itself. The connection needs both an origin and an endpoint. We trace the energy threads as we move through the form, from the inner source to the perimeter of the circle. The perimeter returns energy with resonance. We trace the shape of the phrase with our arms, spinning the silk of energy outward, then reeling it back inward to gather and restore itself.

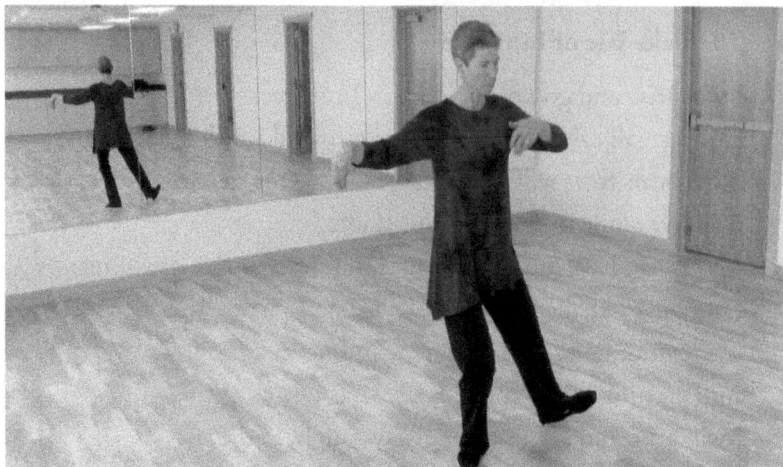

The body transforms the metaphor of spinning silk into a line of energy.

The relaxed, lively, and supple fingers softly come together to indicate the bird's beak. The muscles exert just enough effort to keep that long, conical shape. The thumb stays straight and simply touches the rest of the fingers wherever it lands; the fingers don't come up to meet it. Because this very specific shape is created many times, it can be a kinesthetic reflection on precision, clarity, and a "less is more" approach to movement.

The cupped left hand is shaped to hold a pool of nectar, rising up to the bird's beak. Then the bird, hovering above, takes a symbolic sip. Now, both arms move out – first the top hand, then the cupped bottom hand. Follow the "whip" with your eyes and allow the gaze to expand outward beyond the hand.

The foot positioning grounds you on a wide base, to rest in a comfortable, solid, and stable stance at the end of the phrase. A neutral knee makes for smooth, easy travel out to the left side.

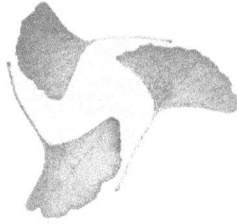

Chapter 3

Brush Knee and Push Step

Symbolism, Tradition, and Background

"Peaceful Harmonious Fist" is my favorite English translation of t'ai chi ch'üan. At first glance, the words seem contradictory. On reflection, they convey the idea of energy contained and delivered in a powerful yet relaxed way. In my life, I cherish peace, balance, and harmony. The practice of t'ai chi ch'üan connects me with all three. For many of my students, stability is especially important, and many have expressed hope that t'ai chi will help them improve their balance.

In a biomechanical sense, "good" balance consists of stability, confidence, and agility. Of course, muscular strength supports these qualities, but it is not the end-all and be-all. We can also support our physical balance by drawing on the reflective, meditative aspect of t'ai chi to invite harmony and balance in the whole self.

For example, consider the yin-yang symbol. Each side of the circle is equally weighted. The elements are distinct, yet they interact with each other. As the yang side wanes, the yin side waxes, and vice versa. The two smooth tails of black and white taper to a fine line, but they don't disappear. The rolling curves of white and black widen to their maximum size, yet they are proportional within the roundness of the whole circle.

Through the practice of t'ai chi, we experience the body's natural ability to remain in balance through the constant cycling of change. Our bodies are dancing to the rhythm of yin and yang energy.

The yin-yang (taijitu) symbol is ancient and powerful, as noted in the following commentary.

Taijitu is a Chinese symbol that represents the interconnection of two opposites. The philosophy behind the Taijitu symbol is over 3,500 years old, and was first introduced during the ninth century, in a text titled "I Ching" or "Book of Changes." The text talks about cosmic duality and the importance of achieving balance between two halves in order to create a perfect whole. The symbol itself, however, emerged much later during the Song Dynasty (960-1279 AD).

The symbol is made up of a circle divided into two halves by a curved line. One half is white with a black dot in the center, while the other half is black with a white dot in the center. The black half represents the yin (feminine) and various other elements, while the white side, known as yang (masculine), represents opposing concepts. Together, yin and yang create opposing but complementary pairs – demonstrating the interplay [of] opposites.[1]

The Dao of Taijiquan expresses it similarly. "Yin and yang are complementary opposites that unite to form a whole. They are opposite in nature, yet there is a harmonious relationship between them; you must have one to have the other."[2]

Often, the movements demonstrate the dynamic and changing nature of weight relationships. Consider the posture of Open the Bird's Wing. The imaginary plumb line drops straight down from the top of the head, through the center of the body, and to the ground below. The right foot holds all the weight and the empty left foot rests lightly. The right hand extends up to the sky and the left hand is grounded with the palm facing the earth. Left arm, right arm, left leg, and right leg all act in dynamic opposition to each other, while symmetry is maintained and the plumb line stays vertical.

Early in the form, several sequences involving Brush Knee and Push Step come after we Open the Bird's Wing. These sequences help us understand and polish weight relationships. One foot steps out, the opposite hand pushes out. The grounding force resides in the other two limbs, bringing stability through symmetry.

The groundedness of this movement is also seen in the combined actions of the hands as they "brush knee and push." We uproot and topple our imaginary opponent with a classic one-two maneuver. Let's say that your opponent is getting ready to kick, approaching you with an upraised leg. One hand slices across the front of your torso to connect with the inside of the opponent's knee, thereby swatting their incoming leg out to the side and knocking them off balance. Meanwhile your other hand pushes out to give the opponent's shoulder a shove. Voila! They're vanquished. Your feet are important players here. By keeping them both firmly and completely down, with a deliberate and intentional weight shift, you stay in a vertical and stable position.

This sequence is rich with possibilities for using intent and "moving meditation" to develop and improve one's sense of balance. The firmly rooted aspect of the Brush Knee and Push Step, with both feet on the floor and the weight distributed in dynamic opposition, tells the body, "This is what ease, balance, and stability feel like." Like a living yin and yang symbol, the body dances rhythmically with change, within a circle whose shape stays symmetrical and stable.

T'ai chi ch'üan is lauded in many communities for its ability to improve balance. In this excerpt from *The Complete Idiot's Guide to Tai Chi and Qi Gong,* authors Bill and Angela Wong Douglas stress the benefits of tai chi for balance.

T'ai Chi was part of a balance study by Harvard, Yale, the Centers for Disease Control and Prevention, Washington University School of Medicine, and Emory University. T'ai Chi practitioners fell and injured themselves only half as much as those practicing other balance training. This is an amazing finding that can change the lives of older Americans.

Although you may not be in the age group likely to suffer serious injury from falling, we can all benefit greatly by having better balance. Better balance puts much less stress on the body throughout the workday, and as tai chi practice improves your balance, you will find that you have much more energy.

Compared to the best balance training in the world, T'ai Chi is about twice as effective. Some of the other balance exercises studied in the Ivy League study on balance were very expensive computer models that required participants to go into a lab and practice. The simple exercises of T'ai Chi are not only much more effective than the other exercises, but they are very cheap![3]

The concept of rootedness is vital when one is seeking to improve balance. But to encourage the light, nimble, and smooth movements from a rooted position, think also of being suspended from above, with space surrounding all the joints of the body.

In *Master Cheng's Thirteen Chapters On T'ai Chi Ch'üan,* Cheng Man-Ch'ing, one of Yang Chengfu's students, conjures up a childhood memory while offering some insight on freedom of movement. This can be applied specifically to the Brush Knee and Push Step sequence:

When Pushed One Does Not Topple, Like the Punching Bag Doll. The whole body is light and sensitive, the root is in the feet...

The punching bag doll's center of gravity is located at the very bottom. This is what the T'ai-chi ch'üan classics describe as, "When all the weight is sunk on one side there is freedom of movement; with double-weightedness [weight on both feet] there is inflexibility"...the energy of the whole body, one hundred per cent of it, should be sunk on the sole of one foot. The rest of the body should be calm and lighter than swan's down. In this way one can never be toppled.[4]

The punching bag doll finds its equilibrium through its heaviness at the bottom. In this same way, our foot placement acts as a stabilizer for both mind and body, nurturing balance and easing the fear that sometimes comes from feeling wobbly and disconnected.

To further strengthen the connection to the ground, Gerda Geddes describes its importance in *Looking for The Golden Needle*. She notes that the parallel stepping allows for stability and promotes the idea of rootedness while remaining light and relaxed.

Walking on parallel lines, be it forward, backwards or sideways, greatly benefits the back because it enables you to 'drop your pelvis' whereby tension in the small of the back is released.[5]

This explanation highlights another way that the Brush Knee and Push sequence invites ease and healthful movement to support well-being. "Dropping the pelvis" helps us deepen the habit of moving from the *dan tien*. This is a term for a specific place in the center of the body, around 1½ inches below the navel and around the same distance inward from the surface of the body. It acts as a power center, turning like the hub of a wheel, which directs energy, or chi, out to your extremities. Therefore, when we drop the pelvis, we create more space and ease of movement around the joints and allow the energy wheel – the *dan tien* – to turn more freely and efficiently.

In *T'ai Chi Classics,* an illustration of the *dan tien* shows its relationship to the pelvis and spine. Viewed from the side, the turning wheel is cradled behind and below, but with a little space to allow for movement. Three important principles are present in that simple drawing: moving from the *dan tien*; creating an open, spacious intent; and inviting the body's components to work together.

Yang Chengfu, in *The Essence and Applications of Taijiquan,* also suggests that we unify the body parts and add intent in order to bring balance and confidence. Here, he describes some nuances of Brush Knee and Push Step.

> Sink the shoulders and drop the elbows. Seat the wrists, and loosen the waist into the forward advance. The expression of the eyes also accords with the forward motion. Push *[an]* forward toward the opponent's chest. The body and hands, each part must unite to produce one energy *(he cheng yi jin).* The intention also extends boldly forward. This will ensure success.
>
> …The term used for the mental intent that extends "boldly" forward is *yangchang,* which implies a proud bearing, with the head held high.[6]

Thus, with the Brush Knee and Push Step sequence, the practitioner can connect with the yin/yang symbol and its meanings of dynamic opposition, symmetry within change, and overall balance and harmony.

Narrative/Lived Experience

Resilience can be a byproduct of big change – if we're lucky enough to recognize it. In 2020, I had a chance to put that theory to the test.

January 2020 began with a long-awaited trip to the beautiful island of Kauai, situated at the northwestern end of the curving Hawaiian Islands archipelago. Birdsong, gentle breezes, and luxuriant vegetation were the backdrop for morning t'ai chi on the lanai.

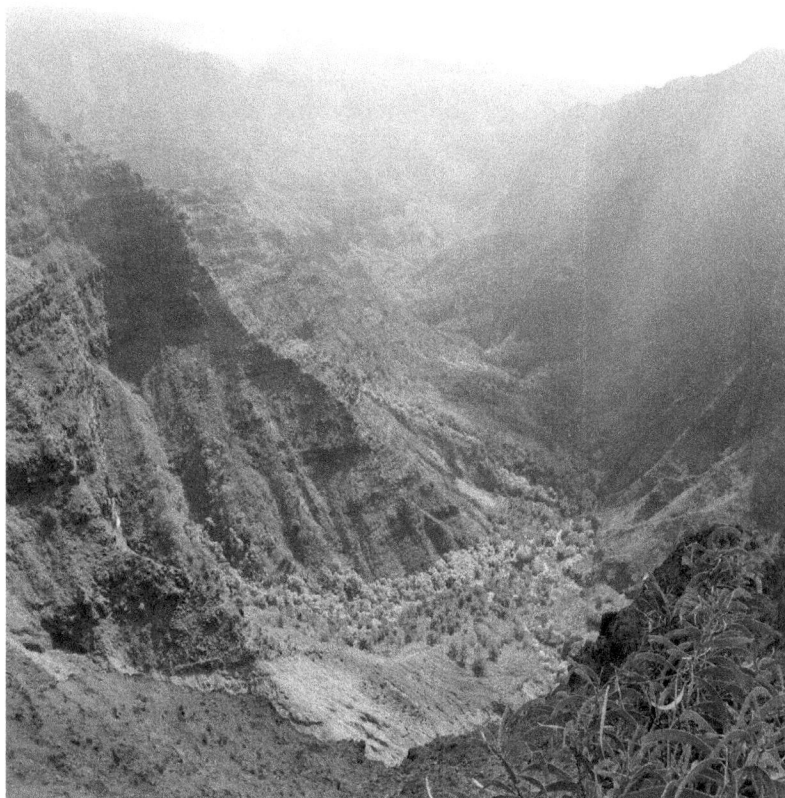

A beckoning landscape in Kauai

On that trip, all my expectations were met or exceeded, except for my plan to keep a trail journal, drawing sketches and writing nature insights while walking on beautiful, winding paths through paradise. It had been rainier than usual in the weeks just before our visit, so the famous sticky, terra-cotta colored Kauai mud was abundant on the trails. It was all I could do to stay vertical, let alone sketch and write.

And when it came to actually getting to a destination – forget it. That idea went out the window one day after a quarter-mile of rigorous mud hiking took us the better part of an hour. We gave up and made our way back to the trailhead. At that spot sat a big pile of walking sticks. We hadn't noticed them on the way in. If we had, we might have gotten the message the sticks were sending: Take one of us, or proceed at your peril!

From rainforest mud to breathtaking views to beautiful beaches, Kauai was love at first sight. But shortly after the end of the trip, life took some strange turns. First, I developed a respiratory illness, followed by pneumonia. Unbeknownst to me, I had contracted an early case of COVID. After that came a late-January hospitalization of my 92-year-old father, followed by his death on March 2, 2020. Later that same week came the pandemic shutdown.

The routines of "normal" life fell like dominoes. I started planning a memorial service and that soon became unfeasible. My two t'ai chi teaching jobs came to an end. Everyone scurried into safe spaces…for how long, no one knew.

Later that spring, it was apparent that this was going to last a while. Early in the month of May, a long-time student emailed me to see if it was possible to meet for t'ai chi in a nearby park. The idea terrified me. On the other hand, it felt good to think that I could be of service to myself and maybe a few others in the community. So we started a little group that has been meeting in the same spot every week since then.

The first meeting felt typical of a pandemic outing. We had joy with a little seasoning of fear, uncertainty with a little courage sprinkled in. In a way, we were connecting with Yang Chengfu's advice – to send our intention extending boldly forward to ensure success.

From our chosen spot in the park we face north, toward a couple of big pine trees. We turn west to Grasp the Bird's Tail, then east for the second sequence of Part One, with its five repeats of the Brush Knee and Push step. We face east for some of the most clear, challenging, and powerful movements: Single Whip, Snake Creeps Down, Fan Out Through the Back, and more. They all require solid, strong feet on the ground.

Our park group usually starts out with a quick warmup and maybe some attention to our feet, especially what's beneath them. Outdoor t'ai chi practice offers many reminders that change is constant: Undulations of the surface, texture, color, and patterns all change on every visit. And as I keep telling myself, resilience is a byproduct of change.

The Brush Knee and Push Step has specific moves designed to un-balance and knock over an attacker – imagined or not – while we stay vertical. We focus our minds and move our bodies with intent, so as to be agile, stable, and rooted. The intent is everything, and then we take that first step with confidence and trust as we step out into our shifty, quicksandy world.

Reflections of Mind, Body, and Intent

Balance encompasses many things: equilibrium, body awareness, confidence, efficiency of motion, stability, harmony, and more. Gerda Geddes offers this insight on balance in *Looking for The Golden Needle*.

> In order to find this balance we have to train and strengthen our muscles. Having a basic knowledge of anatomy is a help, as it is then easier to visualise how the muscles move the bones into successive positions and appropriate alignments, and how the muscles can be used in the most efficient and economical way. We begin to understand how each movement is related to the in-breath and the out-breath and also to the Yang and Yin. When we find the true balance, each movement requires less effort and can be used with better effect. In this way energy can be saved.[7]

That last sentence speaks to an idea that gave birth to t'ai chi many centuries ago – observing the grace and efficiency of the movements of animals. This can deepen our understanding of how the body, mind, and spirit can find balance and harmony with the natural world.

We draw on the components of breathing and efficient movement when we encounter and defeat our "imaginary opponent" in the Brush Knee and Push Step. The smooth, slow parallel step forward with the right foot is in dynamic opposition with the smooth, slow movement out with the pushing left hand. And with the completion of each step, the body is rooted, relaxed, and upright, representing Yang Chengfu's ideal – each part united and extending boldly forward.

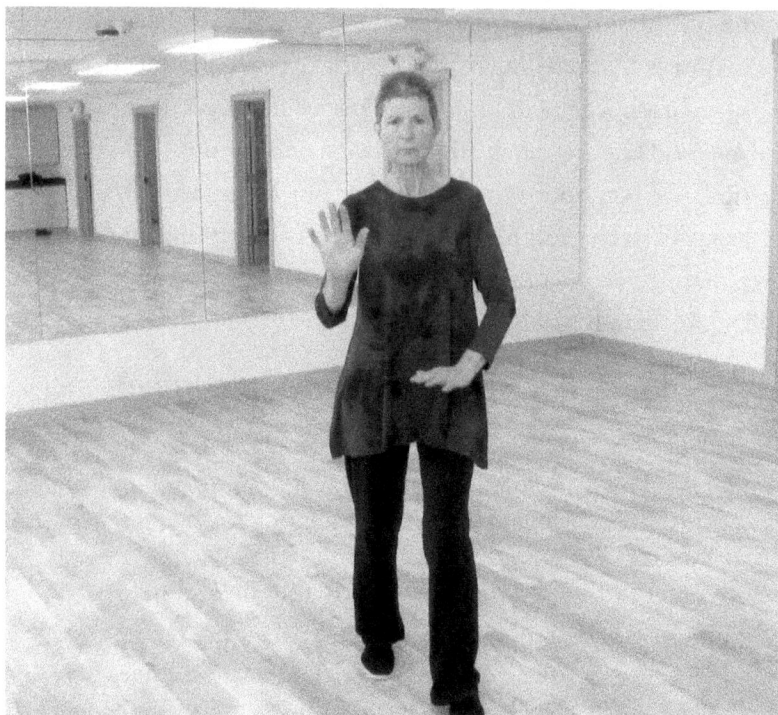

Brush Knee and Push feels symmetrical, grounded, and stable.

Balance is easier if we keep light and nimble. In Part One we have a series of Brush Knee and Push steps, interspersed with a movement called Play the Lute. The hand position for Play the Lute suggests plucking the strings of a Chinese lute, or pipa. The fingers on both hands are diagonally extended upward and softly curved in, as if they were hovering above the tone holes on a clarinet or recorder.

From the Lute position, the hands shift easily to Brush Knee and Push. Both hands move from the center to form a small circle next to the hip. Then, the lower hand pushes, destabilizing the imaginary opponent, whose leg is raised for a kick. The upper hand slices across the body, landing on the opponent's kicking leg to knock them over. By contrast, you stay completely rooted and stable as you step out in parallel, feet hip distance apart, hips and shoulders wide and relaxed, and the two hands moving in symmetrical, dynamic balance.

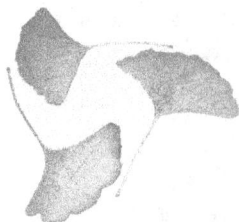

Chapter 4

Repulse the Monkey Thoughts

Symbolism, Tradition, and Background

The notion of "monkey thoughts" is familiar in many minds and cultures. The circumstances vary, but three things are certain in everyday life: Distractions are inevitable, they keep coming back, and it's helpful to keep them at a distance.

In this sequence, the movements and intent represent our effort to repulse those noisy, grabby monkeys, which are constantly leaping around and competing for our time and attention.

We don't try to directly block or destroy the monkeys. Rather, we use our energy wisely and efficiently to deter them from grabbing and holding. Dr. Yang, Jwing-Ming offers this description of the sticky, clingy monkey energy in *Tai Chi Chuan Classical Yang Style*.

The Chinese name of this form is "dao nian hou." Dao means to move backward, nian means to repel or drive away, and hou is monkey. Monkeys specialize in grabbing and sticking. The name of this form tells you that it is used when someone is trying to grab your hands or arms and you are moving backward and fending him off." (Dr. Yang, Jwing-Ming, 1999, page 227)[1]

Here is Yang Chengfu's description of "Step Back Dispatch Monkey" in _The Essence and Applications of Taijiquan_:

From the preceding posture, suppose an opponent firmly grasps my left wrist or forearm with his right hand, and also use his left hand to lift my right fist. Hence I am initially under his control. Just when it seems I can't display my skill, I immediately rotate my left palm up, and using sinking energy (chenjin), loosening my waist and kua, draw it back toward the left rear. The left foot also retreats a step, bending at the knee and sitting solid. The right foot changes to empty, then the opponent's gripping strength is suddenly lost. The right hand simultaneously separates and opens to the rear, and at the point when he loses his gripping strength, immediately pushes forward. Although this form retreats a step, it can still dispatch the opponent's energy. Hence it is named Step Back Dispatch Monkey. Its essentials are in particular the loosening of the shoulders (song jian) and the sinking of the qi.

Translator's comments: "...The word _dao_ [in the form's name, _dao nian hau_] can mean to 'to back up,' 'reverse', or 'invert,' but it can also mean 'contrary to expectation.' Hence the statement, 'Although this form retreats a step, it can still dispatch the opponent's energy.' One is reminded of the English phrase "to turn the tables" on someone.

Note the careful explanation of the timing involved. It is just at the point where the opponent "loses his gripping strength" that one applies the push.[2]

Yang Chengfu's commentary tells us how to outwit the monkey and deflect its energy simply by not being where the monkey expects us to be.

In *Looking for The Golden Needle*, Gerda Geddes also frames this movement in the context of self-defense.

The Monkey Fairy, in Chinese mythology, represents human nature, and, although human nature is basically good, the monkey is very easily tempted into whatever distractions may come across its path. In China they talk about "Monkey Thoughts" which go flashing through your brain.

Whenever you want to concentrate or be still, these monkey thoughts come in to disturb you, so you have to push them away to become clear. Repulsing the monkey is also the essence of the self-defence aspect of the T'ai-chi Ch'üan. By stepping back, or yielding, you can make your opponent lose his balance, and you will easily topple him over, without using force, just by not being there.[3]

In *The Essence of T'ai Chi Ch'uan* we find this pithy insight within The Song of Hand Pushing.

Let others attack with great force; use four ounces to deflect a thousand pounds.[4]

Narrative/Lived Experience

One of my favorite things about teaching is when students tell me how their lives have benefited from t'ai chi. When I teach Repulse the Monkey Thoughts, I usually start by briefly describing the symbolism behind the movements. This brings smiles of recognition. Everyone has experienced the impact of those monkey thoughts, and everyone has tried in their own way to get rid of them. When we repulse them, we gently deploy the t'ai chi ch'üan to meet the challenge of distraction without becoming exhausted by the effort. The five repetitions of the posture remind us to be attentive, fine-tune the movements through practice, and above all, to be patient with ourselves.

From my experience, distractions are not an *if*, but an everyday *when*. This sequence offers a practical, effective, and energy-conserving strategy to send them away – as Gerda Geddes says, "without using force, just by not being there."[5]

It's gratifying to know that I can meet the chaotic force of distraction by merely sinking back and dissolving into the surrounding landscape. That knowledge alone is an antidote to the scatteredness and discouragement I sometimes feel when monkey thoughts approach.

Since this happens every day, I'll choose some everyday events in my own lived experience.

Nacia, a much loved and recently departed kitty companion, had a favorite and goofy routine that she performed every day of her 10 years – trying to catch her own tail. Out of the corner of my eye, I'd see her body whirling – first clockwise, then counterclockwise, trying to pin down that wriggling tail that was always just out of reach. Then she'd give up and charge through the house and down the stairs, paws drumming in a crazy cat rhythm. Finally she would come to rest on her favorite perch on a ground-level window sill. Her body would slowly settle in, breathing slowing, tail still twitching, but thankfully out of her visual range. This usually happened in the morning, right around the time I was settling in at my desk and trying to repulse my own monkey thoughts. It was impossible not to laugh at her antics. She was the embodiment of monkey energy in cat form.

I've concluded that cats are the best free entertainment going. For a work-at-home writer, they're silly, endearing, and sometimes annoying distraction factories. And like monkeys, they are successful observers, opportunists, and predators.

Cats specialize in ambushing their prey by silently stalking. When we place our feet in t'ai chi, we emulate that soft and easy foot placement. On page 56 of *The Essence of T'ai Chi Ch'uan*, one sentence appears: "Walk like a cat."[6]

I often use this instruction for the foot placement, whether it's for Repulse the Monkey Thoughts or other sequences. This is directly con-

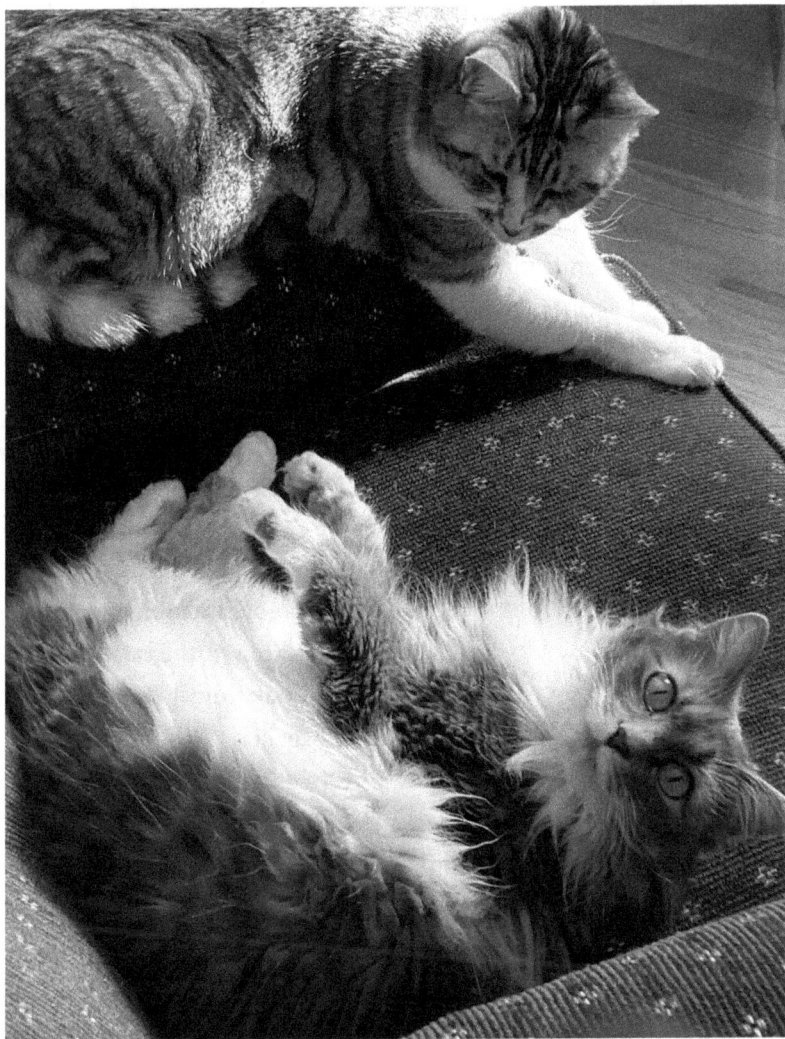

Chief distractors Silver, above, and Nacia, below

nected to the ancient t'ai chi philosophy of closely observing nature and moving accordingly. Cats walk quietly, staying low and flexible. They place their weight with precision, as I witness when a cat steps onto my lap, gently testing the surface and setting the whole paw down. Only then does she shift her weight onto that stepping foot.

With that in mind, walking backward can enhance the grounded-ness needed to deal with distractions. The antidote to chaos is to stay low-profile and quiet, not attracting the attention of the chaos. Move deliberately and carefully, and assess what's underneath each foot before placing weight. Monkeys may dance around, but cats are patient and detached.

Distractions can have a darker side, and these too are regular occurrences for me, at least in the cognitive and emotional sense. To dispatch dark monkeys, I shift into more of a self-defense mode, as Dr. Yang, Jwing Ming describes earlier in this chapter. "The name of this form tells you that it is used when someone is trying to grab your hands or arms and you are moving backward and fending him off." (Dr. Yang, Jwing-Ming, 1999, page 227)[7]

The grabby, gripping monkey has taken hold of me. Now what do I do? It's simple: I must make my getaway. This is where the phrase "Use four ounces to deflect a thousand pounds"[8] gets put into practice.

I intuitively used this method in a frightening situation many years ago. I was confronted by a stalker while walking to the bus stop one morning on my way to work. He jumped out from behind a bush, held me by the shoulders and pinned me against the hood of a car. I quickly rotated my wrists to break his grip and grabbed for the nearest vulnerable body part – his neck. Thankfully, instinct and adrenalin took over and bypassed the thinking mind, so that a small amount of force could hold off a powerful threat.

Years later, I took a women's self-defense class that affirmed what I'd done. We learned hands-on methods to target opponents' weak spots, aiming to disable them enough to get out of harm's way. We practiced various scenarios, such as an assailant approaching from behind and trying to choke us. In that case, we were taught how to exploit the assailant's vulnerable wrist joint, by quickly grasping and rotating it to break the grip.

During the deliberate, graceful sequence of Repulse the Monkey Thoughts, the pushing hand rises and rotates before it extends. That's an exact slow-motion replication of the quick, snapping force that breaks the spell of the gripping monkey. With its hold broken, the monkey energy goes careening off into the space you were just in before you stepped back and dissolved away.

Dissolving means we are not there. We just soften down and away, into the background.

Nowadays, blending in or fading into the background is not always seen as the best place to be. For some, a showy appearance and outgoing personality equals success and power. For others, such as myself, being a "wallflower" feels more safe and comfortable. Whether we choose to be conspicuous or not, the dictates of a youth-centric culture ensure that as we grow older, we become less visible as we lose the attributes of youth.

Age notwithstanding, there's an overall tendency for those who are considered "attractive" to draw extra attention. Anyone in the orbit of the attractive ones can sometimes feel left in the shadows and a little less visible.

Being in the background has benefits. There is space and freedom to know and experience the world around me when I can observe and blend in. This is especially true when I'm out in nature – solo hiking, for example. I find that it offers me a richer sensory experience of what's around me than I might otherwise have if there were companions to look at and talk to.

On a recent hike, while sitting just off the trail on a break for tea and snacks, I heard a couple approaching, talking in moderate tones. I was in plain sight and only a few feet off the trail, but they were immersed in their conversation and didn't notice me. They were startled when I greeted them as they walked by. There's a powerful and somewhat cat-like way to feel about being invisible, or "not there." I can see them, but they can't see me.

As I grow older, I recall my mother describing her experience with aging and that feeling of invisibility. I now understand what that feels like. When I'm out in nature, it makes me feel powerful. When I'm walking down a crowded street, it makes me feel powerless. But wherever we are, and whatever our age, "not being there" wins out on the long run over the monkeys' frenzied sound and fury. We don't need to fight them, we just need to quiet down, dissolve, wait them out, and politely say goodbye to their spiraling energy.

Reflections of Mind, Body, and Intent

The sequences of the t'ai chi chuan are rich in references to animals and their movements within the natural world. "Monkey thoughts" aren't flowing, serene, or harmonious, but they do show up on a regular basis. There is something to learn through observing them without direct confrontation and the potential harm that might ensue from that. When visualizing the movement of Repulse the Monkey Thoughts, we might deflect or redirect them by using a quiet, cat-like patience. This sequence asks us to patiently wait for harmony through the lens of nature.

A meditation teacher in my life often invites students to connect meaningfully with the idea of patiently allowing the mind to settle. He uses the analogy of sand in water at the beach. If I keep stirring it up, it won't settle and become clear. If I wait calmly, it will settle by itself without me doing anything, and then the water will become clear.

Similarly, the antidotes to crazy monkey energy are patience and precision. When we bring smooth synchronicity to the weight shifts and the movements of the upper and lower limbs, we increase our chances of successfully deflecting each monkey. That random energy is met with gentle but firm stability.

By keeping an upright and easy stance, we conserve energy. Ask the knees to stay just slightly bent throughout, so that there is no rising and sinking on the backward steps. Ask the feet to stay energetically connected to the ground below, lifting only just enough to allow a sliver of space while the empty leg slides back. Ask the whole body to glide back as if on a slowly moving walkway.

My teacher Maedée Duprès sometimes offers this cue for the backward stepping in this sequence: "The spine falls back in space." Think about a cat stalking its prey but moving backwards, soft pads landing

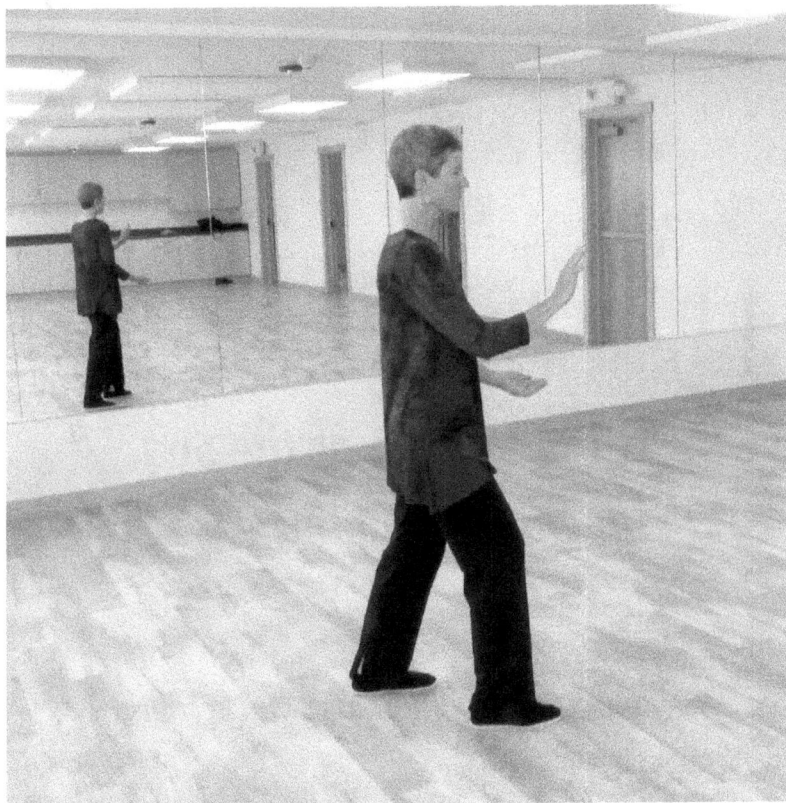

As you move backward in space, you repulse the monkey energy by simply not being there.

on the surface and sensing every fine detail of its texture. Ask the torso to rotate slightly in order to widen the field of energy and vision. Ask the lowered arm to rise out to the side, softly defining the boundary beyond which the monkey cannot go.

Thus, each monkey is deflected to the diagonal, not confronted head-on. As the body travels backwards, it leaves only empty space for the monkey to grapple with, and it wastes no resources on that crazy, grabby monkey energy.

Observe it in your peripheral vision as it careens past your shoulder and disperses into empty space. Then notice more monkey energy approaching from the opposite diagonal, and apply the same patience and precision.

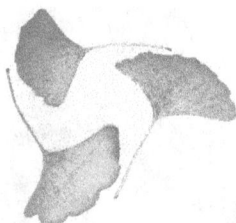

Chapter 5

Look for the Golden Needle
At the Bottom of the Sea,
Fan Out Through the Back

Symbolism, Tradition, and Background

A watercolor illustration in Gerda Geddes's book *Looking for The Golden Needle* shows a diver on a graceful, arcing descent into deep water. The figure is streamlined, clear and sharp, arms outstretched and pointing toward a small and gleaming golden needle resting on the sea floor. A white streamer follows the diver like a vapor trail, bisecting blue-black, cloud-like billows of water. The diver and the needle are tiny elements in the painting. An enormous, light-infused sky and a vast ocean beckons the viewer into a lovely dark abyss.

Look for the Golden Needle at the Bottom of the Sea is the first of the two t'ai-chi ch'üan phrases discussed in this chapter. As we go for the Needle, single-leg strength has its first big test. We summon focus, balance and endurance, remaining weighted on the right leg as we descend for the needle, pick it up, resurface, and then rotate 90 degrees to the right. Then the left leg takes the weight as we step out into a lunge to the left, the movement of Fan Out Through the Back.

By focusing on agility and discerning the path of least resistance, we can flow smoothly through this challenging set of movements. We sink, reach, rise, shift, and lunge – all while gently containing the needle, our cherished creative spirit, in our two hands.

A detailed and lively description of agility is found in *The Dao of Taijiquan*. Author and Yang/Wu practitioner Jou, Tsung Hwa notes that agility, or *ling*, is powerful, precise, and patiently honed through practice and experience. He goes on to describe the infusion of *ling* into one's movements.

> *Ling* is described best in *The Classics of Taijiquan*: "Stand like a poised scale and move actively like the wheel of a cart." In standing like a poised scale, you are ready to react instantaneously. Move like a well-greased wheel, offer no resistance and be able to spin swiftly....Maintain a fluid spatial curve to your arms, hands and shoulders allowing the energy to come to your fingers.[1]

With *ling*, the descent for the needle can be fluid, while the rising becomes light and buoyant. Through practice, one learns to slowly breathe out, keep flexibility and strength in the right leg while bending down, then rise, swivel, and step out. Voila! Yin dissolves into yang, all on a smoothly turning wheel.

Next, the movement of Fan Out Through the Back demonstrates the joy and exuberance that ensues after the accomplishment of picking up the needle. In *Tai Chi Chuan Classical Yang Style*, Dr. Yang, Jwing-Ming offers insight into the movement's graceful extension and expansive nature.

The Chinese name of this form is "shan tong bei." Shan means fan, tong means through or reachable, and bei means back. In China there is a kind of monkey with very long arms. Their arms are so long they can easily scratch their backs, and so they are called tong bei yuan, which means reach the back apes, or tong bi yuan, that means reachable arm apes. This indicates that when you use this form your arms are long and stretched out far, and therefore the jin [energy] is a long jin ...when you straighten out, you extend your arms like a Chinese fan. (Dr. Yang, Jwing-Ming, 1999, page 235)[2]

My teacher Maedée Duprès and her teacher Gerda Geddes both framed these two sequences as a metaphor for the creative force and our response to it.

As Geddes writes in *Looking for The Golden Needle:*

When, in the context of the T'ai-chi Ch'üan, you have repulsed the monkey and emptied yourself of intruding thoughts, you receive a blessing by the phoenix which enables you to **Look For the Golden Needle at the Bottom of the Sea.** The Golden Needle represents the creative force. Perhaps it may also be described as looking for inspiration in one's own sub-conscious. When we find it, we bring up the Golden Needle, and whatever we are able to create with it, we then show to the world in a movement called **Opening the Fan** or **Fan Through the Back.**[3]

Narrative/Lived Experience

Gerda Geddes's insightful description of creativity became real to me about two years into my study of t'ai chi ch'üan. Reflecting on that moment, the 20-year-old memory is as fresh and crystal clear to me as if it happened this morning. It was a turning point in my practice.

About ten of Maedée's students had gathered for a summer weekend retreat at a center near Loveland, Colorado. One of the group members rode up with me, and as we chatted in the car, her down-to-earth personality, resilience, and knowledge of the Taoist worldview shone out. But for the last five miles up to the retreat center, all con-

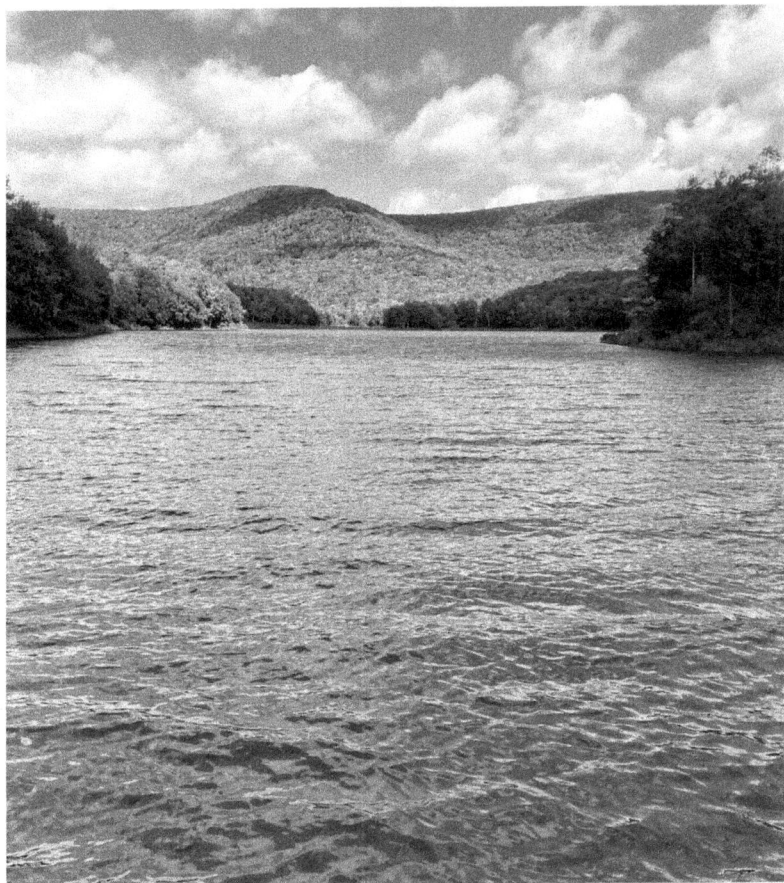

Below the water's surface, creativity calls us. We dive down to find our Needle, then we send it out into the world, toward the distant horizon.

versation ceased as I navigated a winding mountain road in one of the worst rainstorms I'd ever driven through.

We had an evening t'ai chi ch'üan session after dinner in the activity room, and I learned that Gerda Geddes had helped lead a similar retreat there a few years earlier. Somehow I felt a whisper of her presence, like a soft breeze from a distant window.

During that weekend, I studied, practiced and socialized with new and long-time members of a wonderful t'ai chi community. I also deepened my understanding of the movements, tradition, and symbolism. The sessions were intense and rewarding, interspersed with sustaining meals and restful sleep.

On Sunday morning, we had breakfast and one more session outside in the garden. As we did Fan Out Through the Back, I directed my gaze to the western horizon, sending my thoughts out past the extended fingers of my left hand. At that precise moment, a Western Oriole winged his way into a group of trees about 100 feet away. His golden, red, black, and orange plumage, illuminated by the midmorning sun, offered a beautiful and striking contrast against the dark green foliage. The bird's journey across my field of vision lasted only a few seconds, but the cherished memory will stay with me forever.

After that session, we had lunch before heading back to Denver. During the meal, the conversation turned to the unexplainable. Earlier in the retreat, we had attended a session that, among other things, offered some instruction on the chakra system – the philosophy of various energy centers of the body that has its roots in early Hindu tradition. Now at lunch, the lady I had driven up with told of an experience she'd had when she witnessed a chakra physically manifesting in one of her teachers. Other students in attendance at that time had witnessed it as well – a glow encircling the teacher's solar plexus that at first resembled a day-glo pink sports bra under her summer-weight white T-shirt.

This outlandish narrative was told in a matter-of-fact way, and as my lunch companions nodded, chewed, and listened, I realized two things. One, we all witness occurrences that can't be explained or interpreted through five-sense experience. And two, a random or innocuous event can pass by unnoticed, or with a little luck and attention, it can be lit up by layers of circumstance to change one's life.

The lunchtime anecdote, the oriole, and the weekend retreat were lit up by good fortune and auspicious timing. I felt that I had received a clear and simple invitation from the t'ai chi ch'üan: Relax the body, be softly alert to all possibilities of each moment, and keep the sense doors open.

Since that time, spaciousness and alertness to the moment have sometimes brought unexpected gifts. One of these seems to fit in the context of this chapter.

I was in the Colorado mountains with my father, who had a friendship with the caretaker of a big house that featured a spectacular view of the Elk Range. We were invited to spend the night there and got up around 5:00 a.m. The caretaker, absent at the time of our stay, had strongly recommended that we take in the sunrise from the deck. As the sun came up, it touched each mountain peak in turn, like a painter with a brush laden with reddish-gold pigment. At that moment, a big, bright green meteorite streaked diagonally across the sky. We gasped and looked at each other – did that really happen?

Reports of the green meteorite showed up in the local and regional news for a few days afterward. I felt so lucky to have been in that place, at that time, when unbelievable beauty showed up in a random encounter with my field of vision.

An insight from the natural world was the creative spark that inspired Zhangsenfang, the purported founder of t'ai chi. As described in *The Dao of Taijiquan*, Zhangsenfang, born in China in 1247, wandered for many years in the Baozhi Mountains and during that time, learned an exercise called shaolinquan, an exercise invented in the Shaolin Buddhist Temple in northern China. Later, he created tai chi. Tsung Hwa Jo says in *The Dao of Taijiquan*:

> Zhang heard birds on Wudang Mountain making an unusual noise and saw them all staring down at the ground where a serpent was lifting its head and watching upward. A moment later, a magpie spread its wings and descended to attack the serpent. The serpent moved slightly to escape the attack, but maintained its usual cir-

cular shape. The contest continued, up and down, back and forth, several times until Zhang stepped out the door. Immediately the magpie flew away and the serpent disappeared. Zhang then realized the truth of softness over firmness and created taijiquan.[4]

We can't know for certain what really happened to set Zhangsenfang's mind in motion. But nature is, by definition, a force of creativity. It wants to live and move. If my eyes are open to that, my practice will be richer for it.

This plays out in my mind, body, and spirit every time I do the movements of Look for the Golden Needle at the Bottom of the Sea and Fan Out Through the Back. To pick up the needle – creativity – one needs discipline, patience, concentration, and focus. Once it's within our reach, we assist with the left hand so as not to drop this treasure. Returning to the surface, we show it to the world. As a practitioner of t'ai chi ch'üan, and much more so as a writer, the act of "showing it to the world" is simultaneously terrifying and triumphant. Amid the joyous release of a piece of writing, fear pushes in. Am I any good? Will anyone besides me want to read my work? Did a typo sneak in?

Fan Out Through the Back is both a triumphant and vulnerable place, and the body posture reflects that. Arm out, torso open, eyes to the horizon, all indicate trust in the self to express itself, and a trust in a good outcome.

Reflections of Mind, Body, and Intent

When good things happen, it's helpful to remember that luck and timing may have played a part. The reverse is also true. Sometimes, bad things happen due to bad luck. Good fortune and misfortune coexist and influence one's life. If I remember that, I can take the sharp edge off my desire to control it. Then, there is more space to observe and trust the moment. In the movement of Fan Out Through the Back, the left hand draws an arc through the sky. It is expansive…too expan-

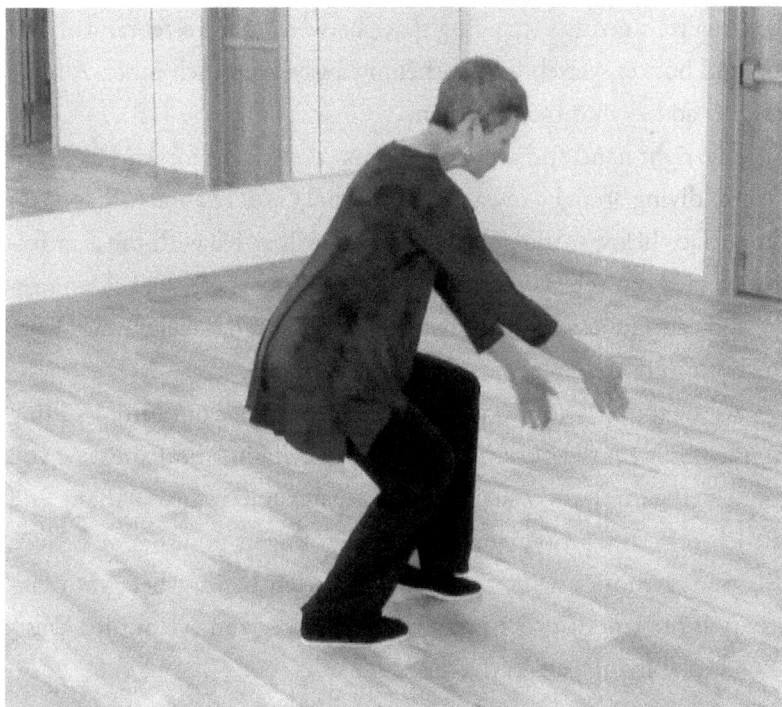

To pick up the needle, the intent is focused yet fluid.

sive to see all at once, but indicating the path forward. Let the eye follow and land where it lands. What is there will be seen, like my oriole.

Fan Out Through the Back celebrates a happy ending. We first spot the needle far below at the bottom of the sea. Then comes the long, graceful dive, the retrieval, the resurfacing, and the joy of bringing it to fruition. After all that, plus a measure of good luck, balance, strength, stamina, and timing, showing it to the world is essential. Let them see it and say what they will! What good is a treasure if I am protecting it out of fear? The expansiveness of the movement lets fear out and trust in.

Throughout this sequence, the body expresses a sense of space. Each gesture suggests outwardness and opennness. On the dive to the bottom of the sea, the eyes focus on the needle, the fingers aim for it, and spine reaches towards it. All of the body extends outward and downward, making itself long for the journey. The hinge at the hip/pelvis connection feels very open and spacious. The spine lengthens when we visualize a gently expanding space between each vertebra, with the top and bottom vertebrae lengthening away from each other. All this space is added with the intention.

The right hand and arm extends out, down, and forward in a gentle arc, diving straight toward that needle. Gaze at an actual spot on the surface below – the point where you will arrive with the arm fully extended but the shoulders still wide. Gently grasp the golden needle and carry it between your two hands while you travel upward from the bottom of the sea to its glimmering surface.

As the torso returns to vertical, the gaze extends outward, focusing momentarily on the beautiful gem of creativity in your hands. As you rotate to the front, the visualization dissipates and dissolves. Then, send the left arm straight out toward the west, fingers pointing out. Now, the gaze extends past the fingertips of the left hand, where your creativity is now on display to the world. And keep an eye out for Western Orioles flying past in the distance!

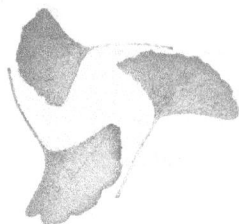

Chapter 6

Spoke of the Wheel

Symbolism, Tradition, and Background

This movement comes about midway through Part Two, and it's repeated three more times in Part Three. The name is enacted by a very specific movement of the arms, in very specific relationships to each other. The right arm is held still and the left arm circles around it, like the outer part of the wheel circling the inner hub and spoke. Subtle weight shifts and foot swivels gently challenge the balance. It's an exercise in harmonizing opposites – full and empty, moving and still. The body dances with those differences as it moves and turns smoothly, like the inner workings of a fine watch.

Gerda Geddes reflects on the juxtaposition of full and empty in *Looking for The Golden Needle.*

Looking for The Golden Needle and Opening the Fan are followed by a movement where one arm is shown as the hub and the spoke of a wheel, and the other arm makes a circle around it. This movement sheds light on Chapter XI of the Tao Te Ching. Here is Arthur Waley's translation:

We put thirty spokes together and call it a wheel;

But it is on the space where there is nothing
that the usefulness of the wheel depends.

We turn to clay to make a vessel;
But it is on the space where there is nothing
that the usefulness of the vessel depends.

We pierce doors and windows to make a house;
And it is on these spaces where there is nothing
that the usefulness of the house depends.

Therefore, just as we take advantage of what is,
we should recognize the usefulness of what is not.

We become aware of the usefulness of "what is not" when we marvel at the beauty of Chinese landscape painting. It is the mist rather than the rocks which gives magic to the paintings. This also relates to our bodies if we think of the arches under the feet and the spaces between the joints.[1]

When the left arm completes its circle around the right hand, it is just below the right hand, which is held in a contained fist with its palm facing downward. At that point the hand opens. The body and brain must learn to be patient while this process completes, so that the fist opens and the energy is released right down into the waiting left hand. We sometimes call this "dropping the penny." Then the left hand moves diagonally upward and both palms face each other for Hold the Circle. At the same time, the left foot swivels slowly to the diagonal, then the weight shifts onto that foot while the body's vertical axis rotates an eighth of a turn.

Now, the stage is set for us to step out into Ward Off with comfort and stability. By attending to cadence, smoothness, and adding a dose of patience, we navigate the subtle challenges of this sequence.

Spoke of the Wheel can be a study in both patience and balance, since both feet are on the ground all the way to Ward Off. In *The Harvard Medical School Guide to Tai Chi*, Peter Wayne examines the science of balance and describes how t'ai chi is so beneficial for it.

Balance is a feat that requires many systems interacting and coordinating in precise and complex ways...Generally, four body systems must work together to keep you from falling over: musculoskeletal (muscle strength, flexibility), sensory, neuromuscular, and cognitive.[2]

Wayne discusses how each of these four systems benefit from the practice of t'ai chi.

The rich diversity of Tai Chi's movements – the sequencing, timing, and combinations of different muscle groups – provides excellent training for the coordination of neuromuscular patterns. Research supports that Tai Chi can improve your dynamic balance as you move and help you recover from perturbations in balance, for example, when you slip on a wet sidewalk.[3]

Dynamic balance is our ability to balance while moving our body, and static balance is our ability to hold our body in a specific position and posture. Spoke of the Wheel is only one of many examples of dynamic balance throughout the practice of t'ai chi ch'üan, but its deliberate cadence and the expressive arm movements allow us to express these contrasts of full and empty, weight shifts, and postural position changes.

Slow and deliberate movements also keep us steady amid "perturbations." Think of a water wheel and the hands of a clock. They turn when they're ready, and if an outside force intervenes, like a flood or the shift to daylight savings time, they resume their unperturbed activity after the disruption.

When practicing this particular movement, we have an opportunity to be steeped in some of the most important aspects of the form. Yang Chengfu, in *The Essence and Applications of Taijiquan,* addresses the issues of calmness, consistency, and deliberate intent.

The most important principle in taijiquan is the value placed on the regularity of movement and stillness. Therefore when practicing, the height of one's stance, the swiftness or slowness with which one extends one's hand, the lightness or heaviness of movements, the stretching and contracting of one's advances and retreats, the broadness or fineness of one's breathing, the attention from left to right or from up to down, the alignment of waist, head-top, back, and abdomen – one must know that for each of these there is a constant measure. You cannot be suddenly high and suddenly low, suddenly swift and suddenly slow, suddenly light and suddenly heavy, suddenly extending and suddenly contracting, suddenly broad and suddenly fine, suddenly turning left and right, or leaning to and fro without evenness.[4]

The great masters, including Gerda Geddes, sometimes refer to the t'ai chi practitioner as a performer. She tells of meeting her teacher Master Choy Hawk-pang for the first time and of his movements that seemed to be a dance of balance and harmony.

The two old gentlemen stood up in their long, gray silken gowns, with black skullcaps on their heads, and performed the long Yang form. When I looked at the 82 year old man [Master Choy's friend], whom I never met again, I had a sensation that he was transparent, like air, as if there was no barrier for him between this life and another life. His balance was perfect, and although he was old and thin, the flow of his movements and the harmony of his body seemed timeless.[5]

Spoke of the Wheel's circles, and many others throughout the long Yang form, all invite the body, mind, and spirit to be fluid, agile, light, round, and constantly changing.

Narrative/Lived Experience

The Space Between

Space and emptiness can sometimes feel uncomfortable; it's tempting to jump in and fill it right up. Think of those drawn-out silences in a conversation when the mind fidgets and ruminates on what to say or whether to say anything. Or maybe an unmarked stretch of slickrock on a remote trail when a hiker's eye is looking out for the next cairn to appear, following that inner compass but feeling an upwelling of anxiety until the guidepost appears in the distance.

To rest in empty space, physical or otherwise, the mind needs to feel safe and trusting. This is not what the mind is set up to do. The website Psychology Today notes:

> To the human mind, uncertainty equals danger. If your brain doesn't know what's around the corner, it can't keep you out of harm's way... you're hardwired to overestimate threats and underestimate your ability to handle them – all in the name of survival.[6]

As discussed earlier in this chapter, the *Tao Te Ching* lays out several ways in which empty space is useful. Here's another: Emptiness can help to clarify loss.

I recently attended a memorial service for a friend who died too young from pancreatic cancer. At the service, those of us outside his circle of family and close friends learned about his life, occupations, beloved activities, and talents. Most of us knew him as a musician and most had heard him play the slide trombone. He and the instrument were one, and this meant he had a gift for nimbly shifting from complicated melodies to improvising in the blink of an eye.

He played with a jazz band, whose members performed at the memorial service. They honored and grieved for him by playing one of his favorite tunes and, in the spot where he used to solo on the trombone, they left a space. The framework of the song was there but the presence of the trombone solo was felt in emptiness.

Afterward, one of the band members described that his sense of loss came through in a feeling of wanting to fill up the space in that solo – and holding himself back from adding notes to the emptiness. What the brain wants to do, the heart wants to do also, and so does the body.

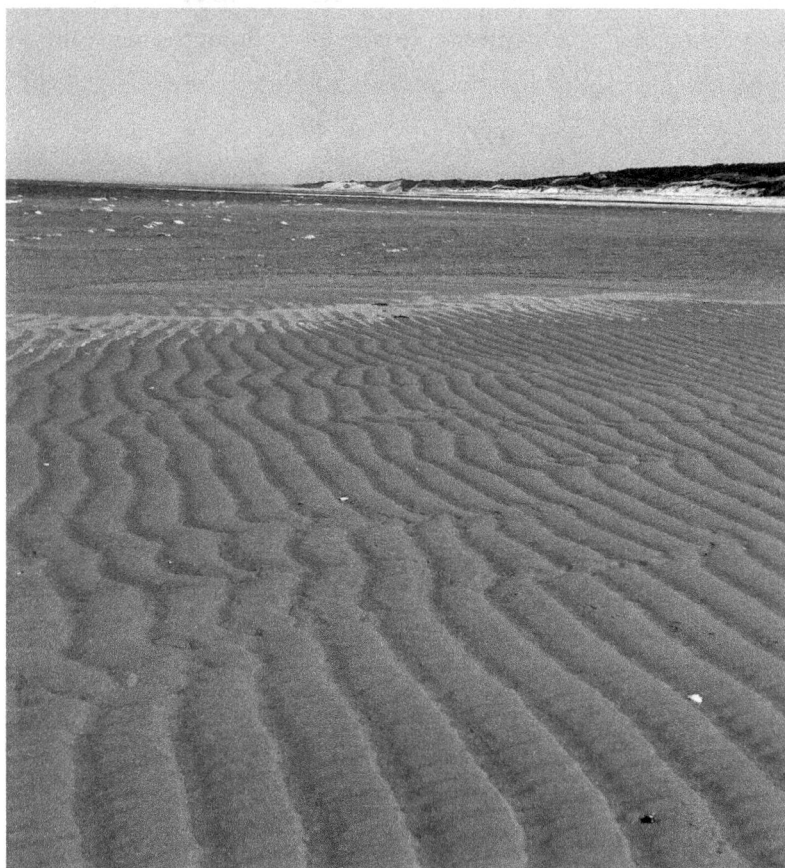

Emptiness, or space between, helps to define life's natural patterns and flow.

Slow and Easy Does It

The movement called "open step" puts us in position for the Spoke of the Wheel sequence. As the body's vertical axis turns a full half-circle, the left arm transitions from the extension of Fan Out to an upraised position with the palm facing toward the face. While the right foot steps out, the arm slowly lowers.

The long, slow descent of the arm allows for a leisurely transition from empty right leg to full right leg, starting when the heel makes contact with the floor. But there is a difference in the length of travel from the back of the foot to the front, compared to a much greater length of travel with the arm, from its starting position above the head all the way to its ending position down to the hip.

There are many places in the form where the practitioner comes across this. We slowly learn to adjust the speed of all the different body parts as they travel through different spatial distances, so that they all arrive at their endpoints at the same time. When that happens, there's a feeling of stability, strength, and celebration.

Sometimes a certain metaphor or symbol appears to help us get better at weight shifting, turning, and uniting those body parts. A while ago, as I prepared to teach a lesson on Open Step and Spoke of the Wheel, I wanted to convey a sense of top-to-bottom fluidity and maximum space between the joints. Creating the intent of spaciousness helps me – and sometimes helps students – to navigate big turns and multiple weight shifts with confidence and ease. Additionally, when doing the Open Step movement, a long, deliberate exhale fits with the slow settling of the foot and the smooth turning of the body toward the diagonal.

To introduce this lesson, I told the students about another name for Open Step: White Snake Spits Out Its Tongue. One student immediately connected with that name. With eyes twinkling, she brought her body around in the half-turn, slowly lowered her left arm and said a long Haaaaaaaaaah! Thus, we witnessed the White Snake Spitting Out Its Tongue. I can clearly picture that moment of triumph and humor. That memory makes me slow down every time.

Reflections of Mind, Body, and Intent

After we're in the ready position, Spoke of the Wheel asks us to slow down and invite patience and discipline. One movement sets off the next in its own time, with a deliberate cadence that is calming and centering, like the breath's rise and fall.

The movements of Spoke of the Wheel suggest that the turning around a circle can't be rushed. The empty space created by the turning left hand won't be symmetrical and round until it completes its journey. When the left palm is beneath, the fingers of the right fist open – like the turning wheel, or the turning gears of a bicycle sprocket. Teeth smoothly mesh to turn the gear, and the timing is deliberate.

In 2000, the year I began studying t'ai chi ch'üan with Maedée, I missed the lesson on Spoke of the Wheel. It was a very long time before I got clear on the sequence, because I tried to just barrel on through the empty space of the missed content. That didn't work. I had to let the gears turn in their time, not mine. My hard-learned lesson was that hurrying past the empty space meant muddying the water and losing focus.

Through the body's structure and mechanics, we dance a narration of all the circles and turns in this sequence. The torso's top, bottom, left, and right boundaries consist of four ball-and-socket joints at each hip and shoulder. Each is supple, smooth, and open, moving in harmony with the hands and feet.

The pivots and swivels of the foot initiate the hip movement. Hips and feet travel in the same direction, and the energy channel of the leg is fluid and unobstructed. Chi keeps the leg precisely positioned yet supple; its unbroken flow creates a smooth, easy movement. As chi

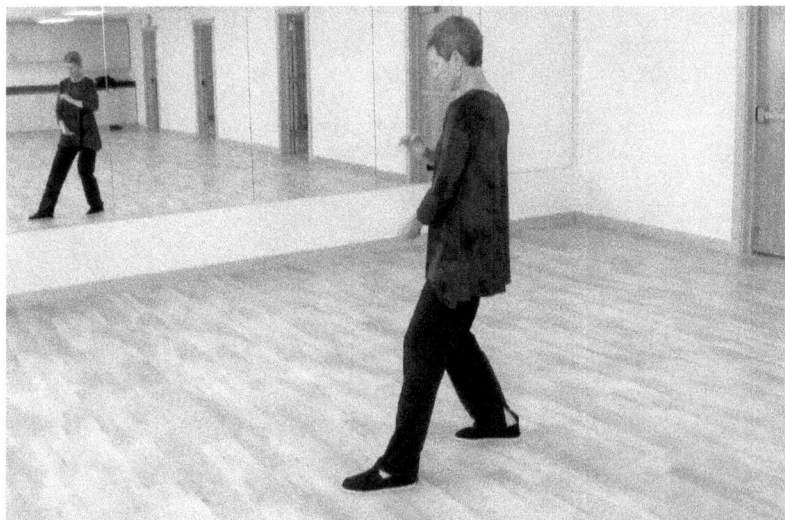

The hands describe a turning wheel – and the relationship of stillness to movement.

awareness deepens, it acts as a balm on any tight or catchy places. The foot and hip support each other – foot adds precision, hip adds stability, and vice versa. Then, the unobstructed chi flows to the *dan tien,* sternum, shoulders, neck, and head.

Chi flow also gives power and precision to the punch and spoke of the wheel. Direct the chi out through the punching fist, then reel the chi back in. The fist is the still and quiet hub of the turning wheel.

The left hand sketches the circle out in front of the body and around the right fist – like the spokes circling around the hub. Slowly and patiently draw the whole wheel, and notice the shoulder ball-and-socket joint slowly rolling forward, mirroring the smooth turning of the hand and arm. Release the right fist, then the hands tell the story of Hold the Circle and Ward off while the shoulders rotate slowly and smoothly in harmony. All parts move as a whole, while the chi moves through its channels with precision, power, and smoothness.

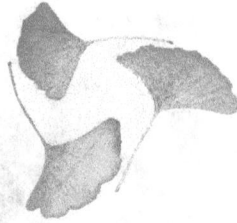

Chapter 7

Waving Arms Like Clouds/ No Beginning, No End

Symbolism, Tradition, and Background

Waving Arms Like Clouds: The name hints at a sunny summer day, when the gaze drifts up to a big blue sky, dappled with clouds drifting in the breeze. This sequence is relaxing and flowing, and students often cite it as their favorite. It's repeated three times, once in Part Two and twice in Part Three. We settle into the name as we wave our arms and move like easy clouds in a breeze, enjoying a gentle interlude just before we perform sequences that feel more transforming, dramatic, and physically challenging.

The smooth, rhythmic exchange of the arms, gentle turning of the waist, and parallel stepping movements invite a tranquil, rested, and nourished state of body and mind. In the allegorical t'ai chi journey, we are hikers replenishing energy before a steep ascent, pausing for a short rest and a bite to eat.

The "cloud arms" sequence feels gentle and restful. Like so many of the sequences, it also asks for patience, balance, and grounding. In *Tai Chi Chuan Classical Yang Style*, Dr. Yang, Jwing-Ming naming the sequence as "Wave Hands in the Clouds," offers this insight, followed by the analysis of the movement.

The Chinese name of this form is "yun shou" and means cloud hands, which implies waving your hands like floating clouds. The movement of clouds can be fast or slow, but it is steady and continuous. Therefore, when you perform this form you wave your hands the way clouds move. It is a long-range, continuous jin application. [jin is generally thought of as internal power]. (Dr. Yang, Jwing-Ming, 1999, page 243)[1]

This form is designed to neutralize the opponent's grabbing. You neutralize his grab to the side and use your twisting jin to make him lose his balance. When you twist your body it must be centered and balanced. (Dr. Yang, Jwing-Ming, 1999, page 243)[2]

With that, Dr. Yang, Jwing-Ming touches on an important point in the practice, whatever the lineage or outlook – the supple turning of the waist to direct the energy. This principle, *sung* (relax) the waist, is one of Yang Chengfu's ten points of practice.

Sung is actively relaxed and easy; not held, but still dynamic. Peter Wayne, in *The Harvard Medical School Guide to Tai Chi*, says:

Sung is considered a defining characteristic of Tai Chi. As a qualitative mind-body state, Sung is variously translated as relaxed, loose, or open, or as a quality that permits the natural flow of energy…One metaphor I use to help students to experience the concept of Sung is honey in a jar. Imagine a see-through jar that you turn upside down and then right-side up again. It takes a while for the viscous honey to ooze back down to the bottom…In Tai Chi training, you learn to let things "relax" downward naturally.[3]

The appendix of Yang Chengfu's book *The Essence and Applications of Taijiquan* contains an eloquent description of the role of the waist. Here is the "Song of the Thirteen Postures."

The thirteen principal postures are not to be underestimated. The source of meaning is in the region of the waist.

You must pay attention to the turning transformation of empty and full, and the *qi* moving throughout your body without the slightest hindrance.

In the midst of stillness one comes in contact with movement, moving as though remaining still. According with one's opponent, the transformations appear wondrous.

For each and every posture, concentrate your mind and consider the meaning of the applications.

You will not get it without consciously expending a great deal of time and effort *(gongfu)*.

Moment by moment, keep the mind/heart *(xin)* on the waist. With the lower abdomen completely loosened, the *qi* will ascend on its own.

The coccyx *(wei lu)* is centrally aligned, and the spirit *(shen)* threads up to the crown of the head. The whole body is light and nimble when the head is suspended at the crown.

Carefully concentrate upon your study. The bending, extending, opening and closing: let them come on their own.

Entering the gate and being led to the path, this must come from oral guidance. To ceaselessly exert oneself *(gongfu wu xi)* in the method is self-cultivation *(zi xiu)*.

If you ask, what are the criteria of essence and application? Intention *(yi)* and *qi* are the authority, bones and tisssues the subjects.

If you want to find out where, in the end, the purpose lies, it is to increase longevity and extend one's years *(yi shou yan nian)*, a springtime of youth.

This song, oh, this song, has one hundred forty words. Every word is true and concise, there are no omissions.

If inquity proceeds without regard to this, one's efforts *(gongfu)* will be wasted, and this will only cause one to sigh with regret. [4]

Soft movement, whether it's meant to confuse an opponent, enhance the chi flow, or ground the whole self in the t'ai chi, is the salient characteristic of Waving Arms Like Clouds. Naming the movement is the impetus that sparks the intent, which then travels to the chi, and then the chi travels through the body.

In *The Harvard Medical School Guide to Tai Chi*, author Peter Wayne says:

> This quintessential Tai Chi exercise integrates movements of the legs and waist with the arms, uses circular motion to improve blood and qi flow to the extremities, and balances the left side of the body. [5]

Wayne describes a visualization exercise to refine the arm movements, intent, and form.

> To help learn the choreography and experience key Tai Chi qualities, imagine your hands are soft, calligraphy paintbrushes...With this pliable quality of movement in mind, imagine your hand is filled with calligraphy qi and begin to paint an oval. [6]

Narrative/Lived Experience

"More will be revealed" is a familiar phrase that could help students to be patient with the learning of t'ai chi. In my experience, learning proceeded much more slowly than I expected. But the layering of sequences in order, and the repetition of learned material, allowed for a gradual accumulation of muscle memory. After I figured that out, I was able to go a little easier on myself for constantly losing the thread when I tried to practice on my own. In the classroom, I got it, but once outside the classroom doors, I forgot it! This mystified and frustrated me.

I began studying t'ai chi ch'üan at age 46. At that time, my professional life included photography, and digital cameras had come into widespread use in the 1990s. As a college student in the 1970s, my classes in photography included learning how to develop film and make prints. That experience gave rise to a metaphor that helped me understand and work through the learning difficulties I experienced as a beginning t'ai chi ch'üan student.

After a roll of exposed film is developed, prints can then be created using paper with a special light-sensitive emulsion. A latent image, formed through timed exposure under specific lighting conditions, is then developed in a chemical bath.

Developing the print was always my favorite part of photography. I always had a sense of joyful anticipation as I waited for the images to slowly emerge out of nothingness.

That memory re-emerged in my early days as a t'ai chi student. The learning process got easier when I stopped fixating on what I could or could not remember. Instead, I related it to the printing of a photograph when, little by little, the image rises from a featureless surface.

This transformed my approach to learning, as it connected me to an extremely helpful idea: By just resting in the unfamiliar, my body could slowly absorb the t'ai chi movements at its own pace. Therefore, my brain did not need to be the controller. Exerting brain-force to try to master a movement was actually a deterrent to learning. When my brain backed off, I had space to rest in the idea that "more would be revealed" with time and repetition. Just like the blank photographic paper in the bath, the image would appear over time, and my desire to "get it" was not going to change anything.

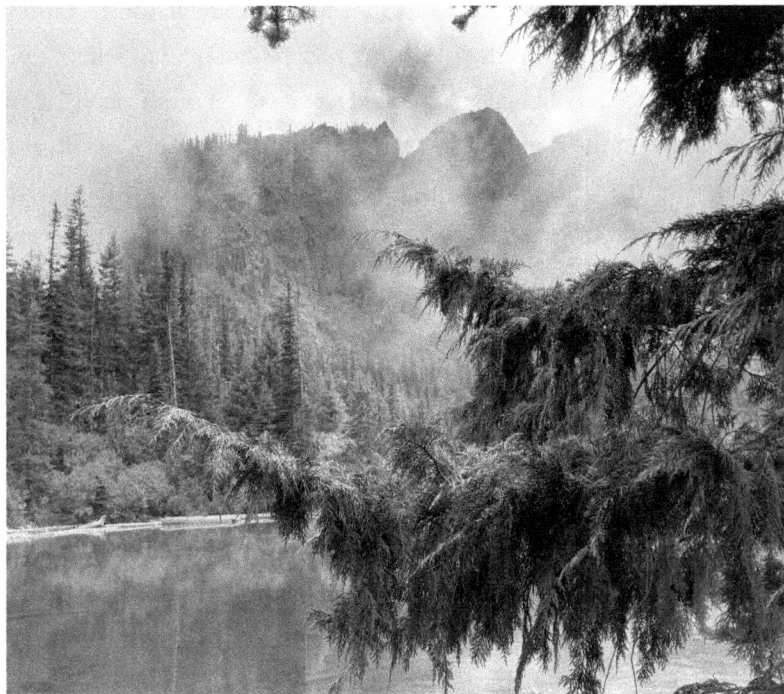

Clouds are ephemeral, and they dance with the substantial.

Of course, my wonderful teacher had encouraged this way of learn-ing all along. But by connecting with a firsthand experience through the memory of the darkroom, I was able to relax more and "rest in the unfamiliar" while learning t'ai chi ch'üan.

The repeating movements of Waving Arms Like Clouds invite the practitioner into a flowing space to settle the thoughts and relax the body. It's a nurturing, healing sequence with the simple foot move-ments and the circular, rhythmic flow of the arms – especially if one doesn't work too hard at perfecting the design. Like the "calligraphy" exercise described by Peter Wayne earlier in this chapter, one can soft-ly paint spiraling shapes around and across the torso, above and below the *dan tien* – with soft eyes that follow, but don't stare.

The fuzzy aspect of the learning process is sometimes discouraging to new students. It's good to remember that this is normal. "Letting your new students know that confusion and directional disorientation can be a 'normal' part of their learning process can help to relieve unnecessary concerns and negative self-judgements,"[7] says instructor Larry Cammarata on the website Slanted Flying: Journal of Tai Chi Chuan.

I try to stress this point to beginning students so they can support each other and offer me feedback without hesitation through the ever-present fuzziness of the learning process. The result is relaxed students and a strong community.

Some years ago at my drop-in t'ai chi class in southeast Denver, a couple began attending regularly. Both were avid learners with medical challenges. One was a stroke survivor who was particularly interested in the fluid nature of the brain. As a retired scientist, he was a joyful and curious student who celebrated the benefits of the practice in his own life. His lovely, soft-spoken wife had balance problems and was preparing to undergo eye surgery. She approached t'ai chi ch'üan with passion and a touch of self-deprecating humor. I was delighted to see her balance and confidence steadily improve.

One morning, they brought me a copy of *My Stroke of Insight* by brain scientist Jill Bolte Taylor. The book describes Taylor's experience of suffering a massive stroke in her 30s and her long, arduous process of recovery. My student, also a stroke survivor, had found common ground in Taylor's story. His own recovery had also been life-changing. Like Taylor, he had experienced a transformation of mind, body, and spirit. Through study and experience, he had become convinced of the value of t'ai chi ch'üan for strengthening and rerouting neurological systems.

In *My Stroke of Insight*, Taylor addresses the properties of the right brain and its sense of community and curiosity.

My right mind is open to new possibilities and thinks out of the box. It is not limited by the rules and regulations established by my left mind that created that box. Consequently, my right mind is highly creative in its willingness to try something new. It appreciates that chaos is the first step in the creative process. It is kinesthetic, agile and loves my body's ability to move fluidly into the world…Freed from all perception of boundaries, my right mind proclaims, "I am a part of it all."[8]

This speaks to our inherent human connection to community. My student had recognized that t'ai chi ch'üan was benefiting his stroke recovery and shared an aspect of that with me. This strengthened my own sense of t'ai chi ch'üan's deep roots in a rich culture, its proven benefits as measured by medicine and science, and the infusion of shared positive energy that comes from practicing together.

Shared energy is hard to quantify. It can't be seen, but it does exist. I can't describe it in terms of the five senses, but I can allude to it through metaphor – especially when someone else's eloquent imagination inspires me. Recently, for example, I read about the release of "Raise the Roof," a 2022 musical collaboration between Robert Plant and Alison Krause. In a 2021 *New York Times* article, producer T-Bone Burnett described the magic of their shared energy. "You know, one plus one equals two unless you're counting, say, drops of rain. Then one plus one could equal one, or one plus one could equal a fine mist."

So we wave our hands in the mist and rest in the unfamiliar. My student who had experienced a stroke and the author of *My Stroke of Insight* had both suffered a catastrophic health event. As a result, their left brains were temporarily offline. Both recovered, and both were able to experience, remember, and take advantage of normally obscured aspects of their right brains. When my student described this experience, he expressed wonder, awe, and boundless enthusiasm for the capacities of human awareness.

If I can ask my left brain to sit out a dance or two, I'm better able to rest in the unfamiliar. Part of that is being "in the moment." It feels slightly unfocused, but pleasantly so. I sometimes need to remind my left brain not to scramble for information and a sharper focus. Many times, being in the moment causes me to lose track of the cues for when "No Beginning, No End" comes to an end. So there's still a need to have that left brain manage, but to stay in the background. Still aware, but softened by that fine mist.

Reflections of Mind, Body, and Intent

This sequence has several names. All of them have the potential to draw the mind into deeper reflection. No Beginning, No End suggests continuous flow, which summons the intent. Then the intent invites the body to move accordingly. Waving Arms Like Clouds might perhaps take us to an open field, beneath a blue sky punctuated by clouds. The clouds could be moving in a stately promenade, dancing past the treetops; the visualization leads to the intent, which then invites us to the movement. For Waving Arms Like Clouds, we steep in the idea of mist and unknown space. The view is obscure, then clear. Either way, the body remembers.

The soft, flowing movements of this sequence are a joy to perform. The gentle rotation of the torso is not only pleasant, but has therapeutic value as well. Gerda Geddes notes in *Looking for The Golden Needle:*

> The "cloud arms" also have medical connotations. There is a considerable turning of the waist and the torso, which gives massage to the liver and the stomach, thereby preventing illnesses entering these organs.[9]

To get the hang of the arm exchange pattern, patience is needed. It's elusive, a little like that old childhood question: Can you rub your stomach with one hand while patting your head with the other? How about walking and chewing gum at the same time? For me, the answer is "sometimes." But by thinking of something random and a bit silly like that childhood challenge, I can chuckle when I'm faced with one of those "Why can't I do this?" moments. Another helpful method is to try to be comfortable with getting lost. I'm always a little bit lost while waving my arms in those clouds that keep changing their shape.

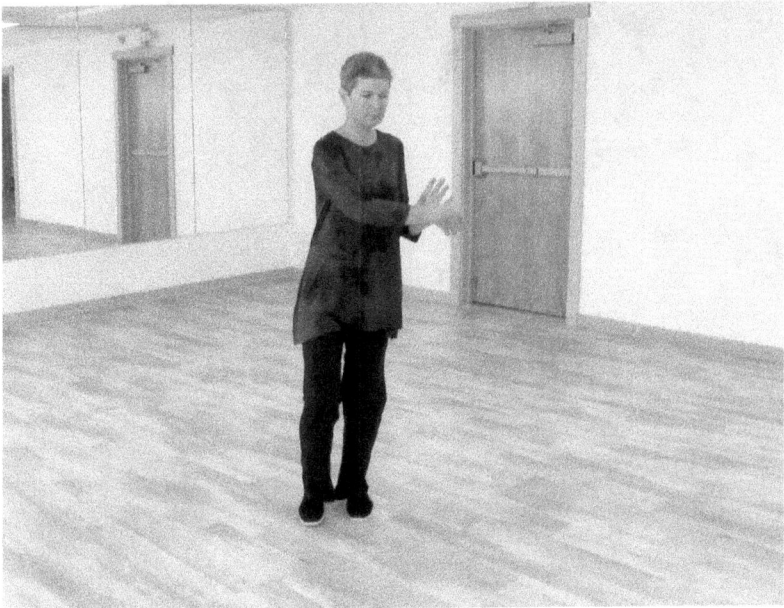

With time and patience, the body catches on to the flow of Waving Arms Like Clouds.

The feet provide a straightforward movement to offset the wavy, cloudy arms. The parallel steps support the intent to completely root each foot, so that the chi and the weight can pour right down into the standing leg and foot. Notice the sinking of the weight and chi downward as you set the left foot down, rolling from inside to outside, with the heel and all five toes in soft contact with the ground as the weight shift is completed. There is a sense of comfort and stability, springy and supportive as a bed of moss.

The hands dissolve out of their Bird's Beak and Single Whip shapes to trace a repeating pattern. One hand and arm scoops down, while the other hand and arm draws across the body. They meet, exchange, and dance in the pattern of Waving Arms Like Clouds. The eyes stay in peripheral vision, so that the head, neck, and torso can softly turn to follow the movements.

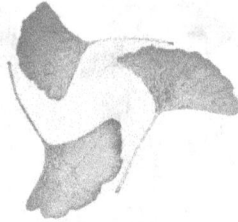

Chapter 8

Full Kick and Turn

Symbolism, Tradition, and Background

The Full Kick and Turn comes near the end of the "kicking section," an action-packed, intense but short series of sequences featuring kicks, turns, and punches. The energy of the kicking section is that of a strong, confident self that navigates the challenges and adventures of life with joy, grace, and equanimity.

Quite a few of the phrase and sequence names in the kicking section are descriptive rather than symbolic. But there is also meaning and enrichment to be found when we connect specific movements with different stages and aspects of the human experience. In *Looking for The Golden Needle*, Gerda Geddes describes her personal interpretation of t'ai chi through the lens of an "allegorical journey."

The T'ai-chi Ch'üan functions on different levels and people approach it in their own personal way and for special reasons. You could be attracted by the self defence part or by its philosophical background, by the sheer beauty of its movements or for health reasons; but whatever way you choose, if you persevere, you will eventually become aware of the various levels, and the T'ai-chi Ch'üan will become an organic whole, entirely your own, with your overtones and characteristics and your own understanding.

In trying to comprehend the *whole* of the T'ai-chi Ch'üan one finds that moving through the three parts and the thirteen sequences is like passing through life from birth to death, from beginning to end, both on the physical and the philosophical plane. One enacts, through the body, the different phases of development common to us all.[1]

The kicking section, in the context of Geddes's allegorical journey, evokes the energy of an action-packed, robust life of a full-grown adult. From that standpoint, we enact that experience as the kicks get slowly more challenging and lead us up to our physical peak where we then deploy all our resources to perform the "grand finale" that completes Part Two.

If we apply a more competitive martial-arts filter to the kicking section, the rapid-fire kicks and turns serve to confuse, befuddle, and unbalance our opponent, setting them up for the coup de grace.

Yang Chengfu, in *The Essence and Applications of Taijuquan*, sets the stage for the left-footed kick sequence by first giving the reader a "what-if" example. (In my own teaching, the "imaginary opponent" often provides me with a clear way to help students make sense of a movement. Yang Chengfu does the same.)

From the previous posture, [Twisting the Tiger's Ears], suppose there is an opponent coming on my left flank to strike at my rib cage. I quickly use my left hand to stick to the back of the opponent's right hand, drawing in, then splitting *(lie)* open. The right foot makes a slight shift to the right. The left foot at the same time lifts upward toward the front, kicking toward the opponent's ribs or abdomen…

…If an opponent comes to strike from behind my back to my left, I quickly spin my body in an about-face to the rear. At the same time the body is turning, the left foot draws in and is suspended in the turn to the right, toward the front. During this turn, the ball of the right foot serves as the pivot *(shuji)* for the spinning of the whole body.[2]

Yang Chengfu's description suggests the goal of staying rooted throughout many rapid spins and kicks. With a similar goal in mind, but seen through a different filter, Gerda Geddes's reflection on this sequence also speaks to the idea of staying grounded and balanced to conserve strength and energy. As she states in *Looking for The Golden Needle:*

The last sequence in the second part is mainly concerned with finding reliable balance in the body by standing on one leg and kicking out slowly…Other movements [in the kicking section] relying on dynamic energy are *Twisting the Tiger's Ears* and *Grasping the Tiger by Both Ears.* Are you in control of your tiger, or is the tiger in control of you?[3]

Narrative/Lived Experience

In January 2006, I was in the early days of a year-long t'ai chi ch'üan teacher certification program with Maedée Duprès and five colleagues. After experiencing sudden and severe symptoms of pain and numbness, I underwent an MRI, which revealed an abscess in my lower spine, later determined to be a staph infection. The abscess ruptured, causing a life-threatening condition: septicemia, or blood poisoning.

During the weeks after emergency surgery and an eight-day hospital stay to get the infection under control, my life force felt like a sputtering candle. The aftereffects of septicemia and a smorgasbord of strong medications meant that, if all went well, I was facing a painful, fatiguing, and tedious months-long process to put myself back together. As I slowly improved, I found myself wanting nothing more than to get back with my fellow students and continue learning to teach t'ai chi ch'üan.

At the time, I had no specific intent to become a teacher. I had a full-time job that was fulfilling and engaging. I'd been an enthusiastic t'ai chi student for about six years, and when Maedée announced the teaching program, I felt drawn to deepen my practice and go to the next level. I didn't know what, if anything, would come of the journey. I only knew that the little voice in my head was urgently telling me not to miss this opportunity.

The program consisted of a year-long curriculum, including twice-a-week lessons, four three-day weekends of intensive study and practice, and a research project. The first of the four weekend intensives went smoothly. A few months later, during the second weekend, I was missing from the gathering and my colleagues were sending me supportive energy as I underwent surgery. A few weeks later, "normal" life was still very far away, but I decided to ask Maedée if she could see a way for me to resume the certification program. She agreed to give it a try.

I scared my fellow teacher trainees when I appeared in an evening session in early February, still hooked up to a tube running to a fanny pack full of IV antibiotics. I was so thin and weak that one of them told me I looked like a ghost. Their concern and support gave me the power to continue the slow trudge on the road to recovery. I faced many obstacles and discouragements and often felt that the self I'd been before the injury was gone forever.

This sequence in the kicking section, Full Kick and Turn, was one of the hardest obstacles to overcome. Just thinking about that fancy kick, then my whole body pivoting on the tiny space of the ball of my right foot – it felt like jumping out of a plane without a parachute. My brain was dead set against even trying it. It whispered to me, suggesting the possibility that if I attempted this move, I could undo all my hard

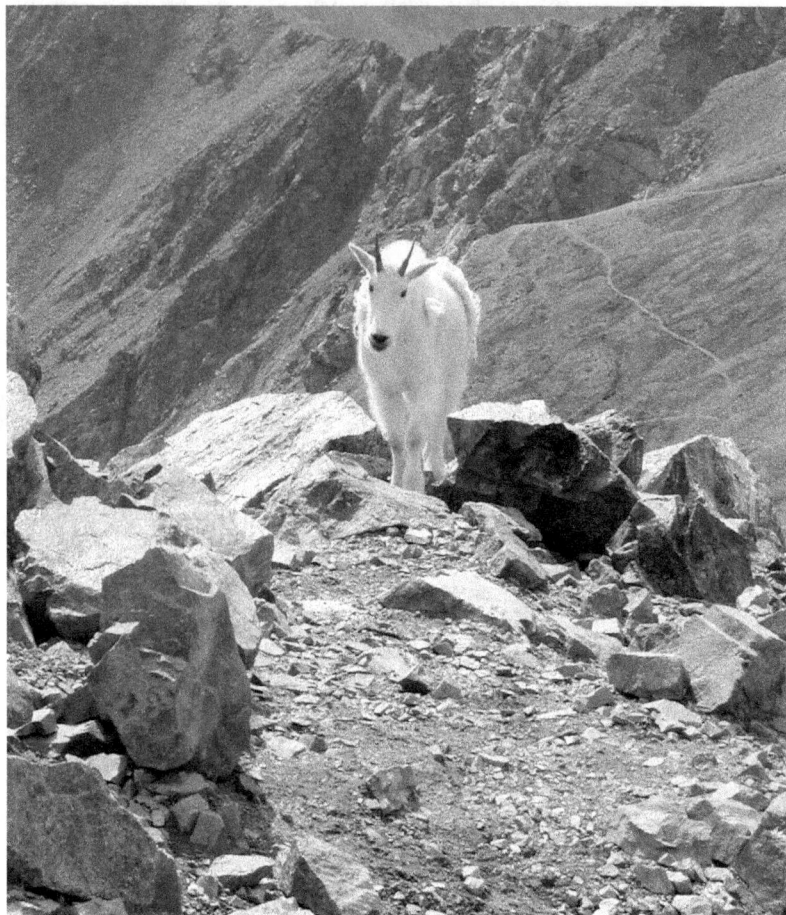

The intent of balance and grounding supports ease and confidence.

recovery work. I might fall down and break in a million pieces, like a wine glass on a tile floor. Fear was my tiger, and it was in control of me.

When I first learned this kick and turn around six years before my injury, I felt uneasy every time I attempted it...especially when my teacher was watching! I mustered my usual coping mechanism of muscling through. I pushed too hard, then spun too fast and lost track of where my body was in space. This meant I couldn't reliably make a stable landing – and if I did, it would be 100% muscle power and 0%

power of intent. After lots of practice, I was finally able to sense the vertical plane and maintain my balance throughout the turn.

After the injury, my impaired strength and balance meant that the kick and turn felt extremely tenuous and wobbly. One day, after shedding tears of fatigue and frustration, I discovered a way to work around the obstacle. It was the ground under my feet, patiently waiting for me to figure out that it had been there all along. As I visualized and placed my intent on the solid ground beneath me, the fear of empty space began to recede and the joy started coming back. Soon I was able to kick and land, my foot finding and attaching to the ground reliably. The sweet spot was the last little movement of the left foot, toe down first on the diagonal, then the ball of the foot rotating an eighth of a turn. The whole foot then descended and my body stayed solidly in its vertical axis.

T'ai chi is often referred to as a "mind-body" activity. During my recovery, it sometimes felt more like "mind versus body." In the act of working through the left foot kick and turn, my brain seemed to have taken on the role of deciding that I should be afraid. It was the fear tiger, and it would not relinquish its power easily.

The fear tiger will never be fully absent. But when it gets too close, I bow and consider a workaround. Direct confrontation is never a good idea.

Sometimes a workaround can come from the outside, in the form of encouragement and support.

I have twice been on the summit ridge of Mount Yale, a 14,199-foot mountain in Colorado's Sawatch Range. The first time, it was sunny and clear, but I turned back before the top because of the fear tiger. The climb up had been pleasant, but as we approached the summit, the pile of rocks felt shakier and shakier, until I realized I needed to turn around. I was with my father that day, and he encouraged and supported me as I crab-walked my way down, crying and trembling, to a place where some soft, reassuring dirt appeared beneath the pile of rocks.

A few years later, my son and I climbed Mount Yale together, and once again I encountered the fear tiger, lurking on the pile of rocks near the summit. This time, we were up in the clouds with no expansive view to orient me in space. I focused instead on two things – a tall stick next to the summit marker and my son's voice telling me I could get there. We both got there, but we didn't linger on the cold, wet, and foggy mountaintop. I didn't shake with fear all the way down, but I did shake with fatigue.

In both of my trips up Mount Yale, the fear tiger was present and in control of my body and my mind – or more accurately, my brain. My brain had done its job – to gather in sensory input and respond appropriately with a fear message. It wasn't wrong. Fear is a natural and necessary result of the brain's input from, and reaction to, our physical environment. Fear exists to protect a living organism from potential harm.

This fundamental aspect of nature also aligns with the laws of physics. When we are spinning in space, we are using our balance – our body's innate ability to orient itself. As the body does its job, the brain gives and receives feedback.

The ground serves a similar function: providing support and feedback. As Newton's third law states, "For every action, there is an equal and opposite reaction."

That is exactly what I discovered when I strengthened my connection to the ground. Its force provided me with encouragement and support on the kick and turn. A vulnerable, emotional moment was mitigated by science.

Sometimes the fear tiger pounces on me in places when I'm not in physical harm's way.

When I taught drop-in classes, on any given day a group might include students I'd known for years, students I'd never met before, students who had practiced for decades, and students who had never done t'ai chi.

New students usually liked to find a spot in the back row, or along the wall. In one of my former classrooms, there was a barre (handrail) along the entire length of the left and right sides of the studio. Several students had limited physical abilities, such as arthritis or Parkinson's disease, so the barre was a welcome support. Others made use of the barre when recovering from injuries or undertaking more complex movements.

One student, Stephen, woke up my fear tiger every time he came to class. He was an elderly gentleman and an occasional attendee who had been a professional dancer, but now was bent nearly double with osteoporosis. His slow walk was almost a shuffle, feet barely clearing the floor as he took his spot on the left side of the room, usually arriving about 15 minutes into the class. He usually wore a pressed white dress shirt, and his trousers, well-cut and tidily belted, hung loosely on his stick-thin frame, with about two inches of cuff dragging on the wooden floor. All of this made the fear tiger claw urgently at my heart.

Nearby students eyed him nervously. I think we all braced for catastrophe every time he came to class. But he persevered cheerfully, following the movements as well as he could. His spine was so bent that he had a hard time looking up at me, and his turns were much slower than the rest of the group. I never saw him touch the barre, but he stayed near it. That's a proven balance strategy, and it also keeps the fear tiger at bay. We may not need the support, but it's a reassuring presence if and when we do.

Stephen also made me a better teacher. In his presence, and in that of others of differing abilities, I learned to adjust my cadence and form, based on who was in the group of students on any given day. I learned to widen my peripheral vision so I could spot the clues each student offered. What challenged them, what brought them joy, what made them tired, what made them frustrated? In this movement, the full kick and turn, there is an invitation to dance with the tiger, taking many "connect the dots" steps around the circle, and as much time as needed, asking the ground to hold us in place along the central axis. If needed, we could simply stay on one dot and wait for the group to catch up around the circle.

From my early days of learning until now, the t'ai chi ch'üan has acted as a rudder to help adjust my mental, spiritual, physical, and emotional course. It asks me to be clear and gentle with what is happening here and now. Then, that nagging question "what if" arises from curiosity, not dread. "What if I fall?" or "What if I don't do this right?" can shift to "What if the arms can help the spiraling energy stay strong and tight?" or "What if the kicking leg relaxes more?" or perhaps "What if I breathe throughout the sequence?"

When the mind and body unite to act "as though" instead of focusing on a specific and self-imposed goal, the practitioner opens up to the three guiding principles of flow, balance, and clarity.

In *Looking for The Golden Needle*, the three principles are named at the very beginning of the chapter titled "The Process of Learning."

> From cradle to grave we go through a process of change, of 'becoming' and 'de-becoming'; we are, all the time, on our way towards something else. The allegorical journey of the T'ai-chi Ch'üan shows these natural stages of transformation with great clarity. According to Chuang Tzu, our starting point is one of original ignorance; we have no knowledge. As we go through life we accumulate knowledge and learning which we eventually have to shed again, so that at the end of our life we no longer have to hold on to our knowledge. Working with the T'ai-chi Ch'üan is a process of learning and un-learning. As far as learning is concerned, one has to adhere to its three basic principles:
> 1) **Flow**
> 2) **Balance**
> 3) **Clarity**[4]

This passage informs my approach to t'ai chi ch'uan as a student and as a teacher: I can't go wrong if I think like a beginner.

Reflections of Mind, Body, and Intent

My brain is hardwired to be more comfortable in the land of what is known. T'ai chi ch'üan asks me to step out of that place and reside in "moving meditation." That means staying in the present moment and not fully engaging with what comes next. Early in the learning process, it sometimes felt as if my brain and my mind-body "self" were working toward two different goals. My brain had the goal of "getting it" – being able to perform the movements consistently and properly and to clearly remember the sequences. My mind-body "self" sought to experience the quality of being in the moment with curiosity and a patient, open quality of learning. But how could I get both brain and self in that space?

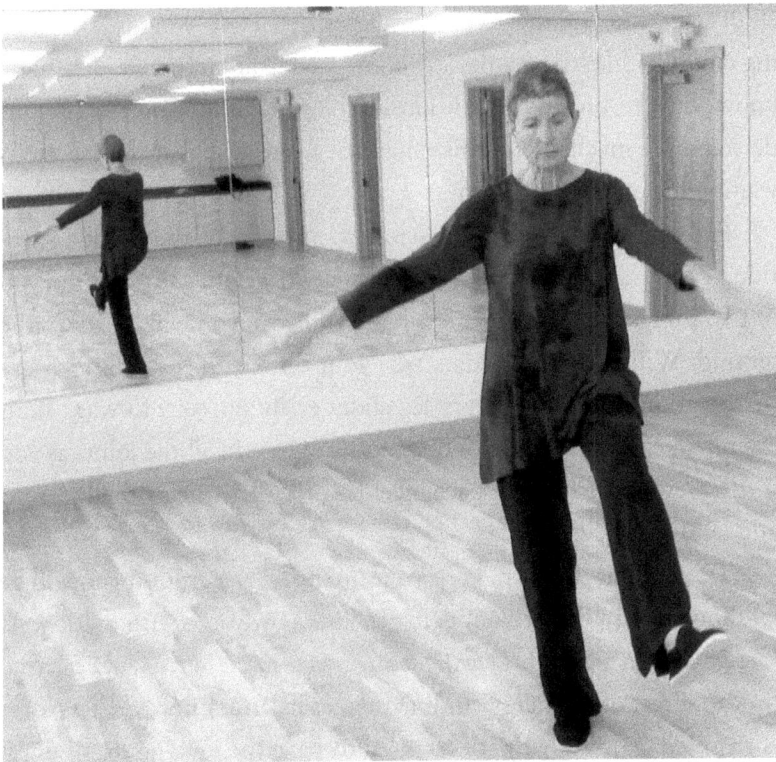

A ssense of groundedness and a stable vertical axis are the keys to the Full Kick and Turn.

One strategy is to involve the breath in each movement, natural and easy, and imagine that the breath is actually doing the movement. Gerda Geddes notes the importance of this.

> When one has practised for a long time, the process of breathing seems to take over and it becomes the most important part of the T'ai-chi ch'üan. In fact, it feels as if the breath becomes the Master and it does the T'ai-chi for you.[5]

Several of my meditation teachers, when giving instructions on the breath, have made reference to the tiny "gap" at the end of an exhale and just before the inhale. For me, this gap seems to be the unknown – not something my brain needs to be afraid of, but just one of the places in between. To be confident in this movement, where the empty leg kicks and then turns through space, I ask "what if" the turning could be like the gap between an exhale and an inhale. My body knows how to breathe, and it knows the gap without needing to understand the mechanics. In like manner, I can trust that the ground is waiting for my foot to return.

Full Kick and Turn occurs close to the end of the "kicking section" – the grand finale of Part Two. The two weight shifts remind you of two things: one, you are grounded, and two, you will return to the ground. With that knowledge, take your time with the kicking foot's presentation. First, the empty leg slides easily out and forward from the hip. Next, find a sense of openness and ease in all the joints as you softly present the foot in space, heel-ball-toe. Then relax the leg, turn and land. No rush.

Throughout the turn, keep your intent on the ground you will be landing on to build the confidence to kick slowly and with fluidity. As Gerda Geddes notes in *Looking for The Golden Needle*, "One learns... how to direct one's energy, finding that, as balance improves, less force is required."[6] That's why it's essential to have the kicking leg as empty as possible. Think of opening the hip without using any of its muscle power to launch.

The arms sketch a circle, which also helps to ground you and define your space. Think of them as stabilizers, like the outriggers on a catamaran that keep the boat's center in its place. Or you could also visualize twirling an upright stick that has ribbons attached to the end. As it rotates, the ribbons softly soar out and then back in to wrap themselves around the stick. In a similar manner, the arms follow the torso as it rotates, with the energy spiraling outward from the center.

Therefore, in this movement we can simply enact the physical laws of nature and circular motion. The chi, spinning out from the center, powers the body around in a circle. We could even say that this reflection is also a scientific experiment in the effectiveness of t'ai chi. We find the ground, and we find where we are in space, solidly rooted on the left side along our rotating vertical axis.

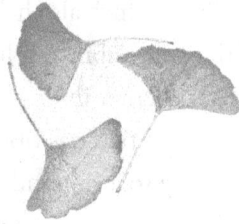

Chapter 9

Seven Steps of the Buddha/
Parting of the Wild Horse's Mane

Symbolism, Tradition, and Background

The two names for this sequence place us in two very different metaphorical landscapes.

"Seven Steps of the Buddha" refers to the story of the Buddha's birth. It is said that, immediately following his birth, he took seven steps in each of the four directions. Beneath each foot, a lotus flower bloomed.

This particular version of the story offers beautiful nature images to set the stage for the Seven Steps.

> One day in the last month of her pregnancy, [Queen Maya] decided that she would like to pass the spring day in a flower garden... The trees were abloom with beautiful flowers that gave off pleasant fragrances; the deep green grasses were like the tail feathers of a peacock and swayed like soft fine silk blown by the wind. The queen took a pleasant stroll; she leaned on the limb of an asoka

tree which drooped down because of the weight of its flowers. At that moment, the Bodhisattva was born, suddenly and yet peacefully. Immediately after birth he took seven steps in each of the four directions...[1]

The Seven Steps t'ai chi ch'üan sequence carries a sense of rippling aliveness. We get that same feeling when we call it Parting of the Wild Horse's Mane, although the imagery of that name is quite different from that of the Seven Steps. The common thread is the idea of a life force that is powerful, flowing, and gentle. In Seven Steps, we have the image of a child's foot, gracefully and tenderly placed on the earth below, then slowly coming off the ground to reveal a beautiful flower blooming beneath. In *Looking for The Golden Needle*, Gerda Geddes describes how gentleness serves as an antidote to the terrifying power of a wild horse.

You finish the second part by **Carrying the Tiger to the Mountain**. It is time to have a rest before one continues in the third part with **Parting of the Wild Horse's Mane**. The mythical wild horse was a ferocious, saw-toothed animal, capable of tearing a tiger to pieces, often associated with the Tartars and the Mongols who invaded China from the north. In the context of the T'ai-chi Ch'üan, one learns the need for great gentleness if one is to approach this fierce creature close enough to part its mane. If your body is filled with aggression and fear, the movement simply cannot be done. Becoming gentle and letting go of the other emotions is part of the Taoist teaching.

It is important to understand the difference between the East and the West in dealing with dangerous, mythical animals. We in the West, in our fairy tales, always have to kill the dragon in order to win the princess or find the treasure, whereas in the East, to kill one of these supernatural animals would be catastrophic; it would upset the whole balance of the universe. The Chinese say that the wild horse, and also the dragon, must be tamed or neutralized. This is achieved by giving them a mate who is gentle and loving, such as a docile mare, and through her intervention harmony will be established.[2]

As we learn and refine this movement over time, the idea of flow, harmony, and gentleness seeps in and radiates out, like the breath. As the body's movement slowly grows smoother, it recognizes, nurtures, and supports the intent of flow and gentleness – and vice versa.

Many t'ai chi masters espouse the benefits of flow and balance – more so than muscle strength. In *The Dao of Taijiquan*, author Tsung Hwa Jou emphasizes softness and agility. He offers these tips to practitioners:

• Firmly root your weight in your feet.

• Control all movements by rotating your waist and whole body without independent activity of your limbs, and

• Maintain a fluid spatial curve to your arms, hands and shoulders allowing the energy to come to your fingers.[3]

The torso brings stability to the diagonally spiraling movements of Seven Steps/Parting of the Wild Horse's Mane. As noted in the description above, strength from the body's center sends out energy to the limbs.

Dr. Yang, Jwing-Ming, in *Tai Chi Chuan Classical Yang Style*, offers a dramatic description of Parting of the Wild Horse's Mane.

The Chinese name of this form is "ye ma fen zong." Ye means wild, ma means horse, fen means to shear or divide, and zong means mane. The horse is a powerful animal, and a wild horse is particularly forceful and vigorous. The name of this form gives the image of a horse tossing its head vigorously and shaking its mane. The word "shear" is used because when you do this form, you "tear" your hands apart as you turn your body. The motion is continuous, extended and powerful. (Dr. Yang, Jwing-Ming, 1999, page 276)[4]

Again, energy spins from a strong and stable central core with the graceful, rippling force of a wild horse's mane.

Narrative/Lived Experience

The name "Parting of the Wild Horse's Mane" evokes childhood memories of riding horseback. At the age of ten or so, I learned to ride, and the Saturday morning lesson at High Country Farms was the highlight of my week. When it rained, as it often did in northwestern New Jersey, I sat by the window, hoping with all my heart that the rain would stop so my lesson wouldn't be cancelled.

Sometimes, the instructor would hold the lesson in the barn if it was a rainy day. There, we could learn horse care – brushing, cleaning hooves, keeping the stall tidy, and how to put on the bridle and saddle. The English saddle rested on the horse's back, just behind the withers, which is the name for the little hump at the top of the horse's shoulder. Forward of that spot, the mane flows down over the side of the neck – a graceful and natural part to the "wild horse's mane."

In my early lessons, I was taught how to give the horse direction, using messages from my legs, hands, posture, and voice. I learned how a horse is trained to respond through all the different contact points on its body and mine. We started slowly – first walking, then trotting. At that point I learned how to post, a technique of rising gently up and down in the saddle in time with the stride. Next came the canter, a faster, smoother, more rippling gait than a trot, which is a "two beat diagonal gait where the horse's legs work in paired diagonals...The canter is a three beat gait where one pair of feet strike the ground simultaneously and the other two feet land independently."[5]

The first time I rode a cantering horse, I felt like I was floating above the earth. That rippling flow of the feet was reflected in the mane,

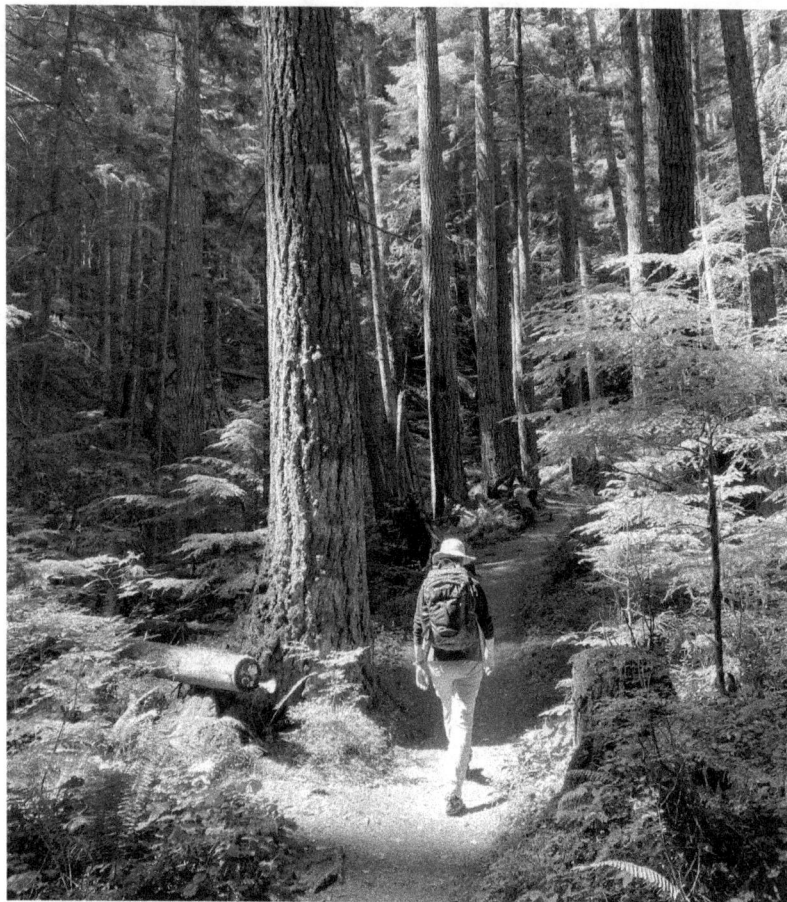

In Seven Steps of the Buddha, we step forward gently in a natural, undulating pattern, as if walking in nature's beauty.

which I saw in my peripheral vision, dancing in the breeze created by the horse's movement.

That's the image I conjure up sometimes, when practicing the sequence of Parting of the Wild Horse's Mane. Soft, floating, rippling motion, with no energy wasted.

A horse in motion is the embodiment of beautiful, flowing energy, and its head and neck move in harmony with all its gaits. The heavily muscled neck assists in forward momentum, and the head, eyes, and ears are also part of the flow.

I kept going with my lessons, and few years in, I learned jumping. In this activity, my teacher and the horse taught me a lot about anticipation and intention. As always, my teacher stressed the overall importance of being one with the horse. Riding toward the jump, getting ready, smoothly clearing it, and landing well – all required me to prepare myself and the horse. "Watch the ears," said my teacher. "When they go forward, that means the horse is ready and willing." It was up to me to facilitate that, and send a message with my body – set myself a little forward, ease up and slightly forward with the reins, maintain contact with my legs, and make sure I went over the jump with the front half of the horse and not the back half. Oof! I did the latter a couple of times.

The forward ears were the most important signal. Thinking "forward and up" is also a way to bring joy and ease to the sequence of Parting of the Wild Horse's Mane. If I am swiveling to the right and left diagonals with seven repetitions, it helps to do those diagonal motions if I keep a forward-and-slightly-upward momentum. That prevents the movement from getting twisted and compressed. It also makes the turning easier, because the forward and upward flow gives space to the joints.

The other name for this sequence, Seven Steps of the Buddha, also brings the intention of flowing beauty and harmony, along with a sense of wonder and curiosity. The concept of a flower growing beneath each footstep asks me to slow down and appreciate the beauty around me. If a lotus flower is blooming under my foot, I would set it down, then lift it up, slowly and carefully. This would allow the petals of the lotus to gradually open in the space beneath each foot.

For me, creating the space for the metaphor is allowing it to unfold. It has a sort of dream-like quality, like that of an actual lily pond. All sorts of creatures live and move among the glossy green leaves with their long, undulating stems and big, showy flowers. Amphibians, water skaters, lily trotters all smoothly traverse the lotus garden. They walk smoothly yet softly, leaving ripples that dissipate within the forest of leaves.

Resting in this metaphor also fosters the idea of gliding with the flow, keeping the footsteps soft. Watching where we place our feet.

We are big animals, but creatures much bigger than ourselves move with much greater stillness and attentiveness to their footfalls. Recently, while hiking in Rocky Mountain National Park in the early morning, I was listening for birds and caught the sound of a couple of small twigs breaking. I looked up just as a large, dark shape appeared in my peripheral vision, about 200 feet behind me and slightly to the left. It was an adult moose, probably weighing 600-800 pounds. She'd probably heard me coming long before I heard her. I respectfully stopped dead in my tracks while she angled ahead of me across the trail. I heard no other sounds except for soft footfalls; she didn't break another twig.

Seven Steps of the Buddha asks me to be mindful of every single footfall. This isn't the same as tiptoeing silently. It's the thought of knowing not just where the foot will land, but where and when it will pick up. When I applied that to my practice of this sequence, it got easier. By staying on the back foot a second or two longer, I gave myself just a little more information about where I was in space – proprioception. Then, the curious front foot steps out with ease and nimbleness. Much is still unknown, but by lingering on the back foot, the lotus flower has a chance to bloom gently as the door opens.

Reflections of Body, Mind and Intent

"Tread softly" is the name of a chapter in *Looking for The Golden Needle*. The rippling gait of a horse, the unfolding petals of a lotus, and the gentle movement of the foot all invite the idea of soft, flowing footsteps. To introduce the chapter called Tread Softly, Gerda Geddes describes her childhood in Norway and the times she spent in the woods with her grandfather.

Although my Grandfather was a big man, he could walk through the woods without making a sound. He would tell me to look at the ground carefully so as not to step on broken twigs if I wanted to discover the woodland secrets.[6]

Years later, she reconnected to this memory as she learned t'ai chi ch'üan. In the same chapter, she writes of her early lessons.

> What my teacher stressed most to begin with was the importance of the foot; how it touched the ground, how each step must be soft and gentle and flowing, how I must be aware of the contact of the sole of the foot with the ground, of the energy which is drawn into the body through the sensitivity and the openness of the foot. Now this was a teaching I understood. It was as if my Grandfather's wisdom was coming back to me through this old Chinese gentleman. This was a language I already knew from childhood.[7]

To infuse this sequence with ease and grace, think first of the soft, gentle, and flowing movements of the foot, with the rest of the body reflecting that light, rippling, ribbon-like quality.

If the rotations of this movement can stay light and forward-feeling, Seven Steps ripples joyously through space. Twisting and bearing down on the rotating foot can leave one with a sense of corkscrewing into the ground, coming to a full stop, then shoving the engine into reverse.

The spine has 26 vertebrae, with pads above and below each one. To infuse this movement with space and buoyancy, I offer an image from the wayback machine: an old-fashioned telephone cord. These cords often got twisted up as we picked up a call, paced around the room while talking, and then replaced the headset. Eventually we had a tangled, loopy mess. The best way to undo them was to unplug each, then suspend them in the air and allow them to untwist themselves, around and back, until the knots eventually undid themselves.

If one can visualize the spine as open at each end, this suggests to the torso that it can unwind itself like that phone cord. The foot swiv-

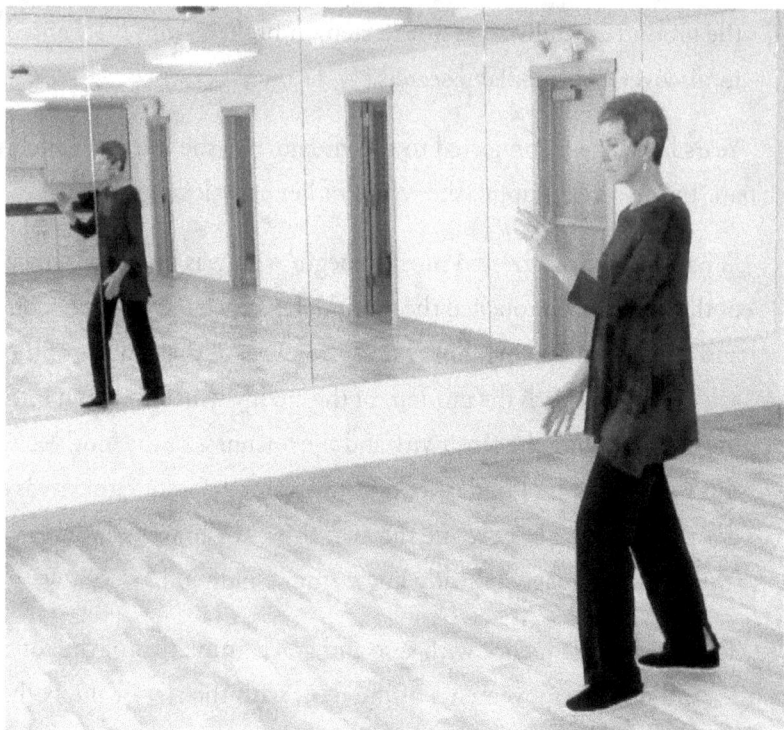

Think forward and upward to avoid getting too twisted up.

els, the lumbar spine begins the turn, then the thoracic spine follows, then the cervical spine, then the head and the energy above. Now, all is smoothly aligned on the diagonal. As the back foot steps forward, the swivel begins its journey to the other diagonal, passing through the center just as the rising hand floats upward and the eyes gaze softly downward into the palm. Like silk, supple and strong.

With that open spine, move the attention to synching up the arms, legs, and torso for a full-body rotation. This takes time and patience. The aspiration is a gentle, easy shift from diagonal to diagonal while the whole body stays tall and carries a forward intention, like a horse's softly rippling gait.

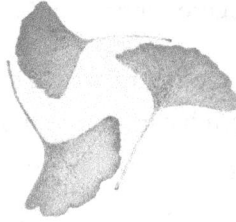

Chapter 10

Fair Lady/Jade Maiden
Works with Shuttles/Four Corners

Symbolism, Tradition, and Background

The Fair Lady (or Jade Maiden) who Works With Shuttles is Kuan Yin or Guanyin, a goddess or bodhisattva associated with mercy and compassion. Beloved throughout Asia, she was first given the name "Goddess of Mercy" or "Mercy Goddess" by Jesuit missionaries in China. Guanyin is short for Guanshiyin, which means "[The One Who] Perceives the Sounds of the World.[1]

"Working With Shuttles" refers to the act of weaving – drawing the shuttle through the threads of a loom in a certain pattern. Kuan Yin's tapestry reflects her pattern of showing mercy and compassion, and her intent to manifest wherever beings need help. We too can intend to be agents of help and healing, and from that point, choose and weave our patterns.

Author and meditation instructor Christina Feldman says:

No matter how hard we try, we can't make ourselves feel compassionate. But we can incline our hearts toward compassion. In one of the stories in the early Buddhist literature, the ascetic Sumedha reflects on the vast inner journey required to discover unshakeable wisdom and compassion. He describes compassion as a tapestry woven of many threads: generosity, virtue, renunciation, wisdom, energy, patience, truthfulness, determination, loving-kindness, and equanimity. When we embody all of these in our lives, we develop the kind of compassion that has the power to heal suffering.[2]

Kuan Yin's weaving is an act of healing and strengthening connection. When we perform Fair Lady Works with Shuttles, we dance to that tune.

In *Looking for The Golden Needle,* Gerda Geddes offers insight on the physical connection with weaving and the metaphorical journey suggested by the movement.

The Parting of the Wild Horse's Mane is followed by **Fair Lady or Jade Maiden Works with Shuttles.** The fair lady or the jade maiden was the Kuan Yin, the Goddess of mercy. She came down to earth to help people in distress, and the T'ai-chi movements show her as working with her shuttles on an upright loom, weaving patterns which will make the passage between heaven and earth easier to comprehend. The Chinese believed that the earth was square, and that the heavens were held up by the four legs of the tortoise whose feet were placed in the four corners of the earth. The movements of the fair lady, through her weaving, are directed into these four corners, and in order to get to her destination she always has to pass through the centre. It could be suggested that, through this sequence, one becomes aware of one's own centre, and that at the same time one discovers the freedom of moving everywhere, in all directions, which includes the four corners.[3]

In *Tai Chi Chuan Classical Yang Style,* Dr. Yang, Jwing-Ming describes how the idea of weaving supports a focused mind and accurate body positioning.

> The Chinese name of this form is "yu nu chuan suo." Yu is jade, nu is girl or lady; together they refer to a fair or beautiful lady. Chuan means to thread or pass through, and suo is a weaver's shuttle. In order to weave a piece of cloth, you must move the horizontal threads back and forth through the vertical threads with a shuttle. As you do the repetitions of the form, your body moves back and forth as if you were working a loom. You have to watch carefully in order to insert the shuttle accurately through the threads. (Dr. Yang, Jwing-Ming, 1999, page 285)[4]

This careful attention to accuracy, he says, has potentially dire consequences for an opponent.

> This form is generally used at close range. From the movements of the form it is understood that you are attacking the vital cavity in the armpit, where a correct strike can cause a heart attack. You must first expose the target by raising his elbow, and then use the secret sword hand form (index and middle fingers) in order to reach the cavity, which is deep in the armpit. (Dr. Yang, Jwing-Ming, 1999, page 285)[5]

Yang Chengfu, in *The Essence and Applications of Taijiquan,* also employs the metaphor of weaving or threading. Like Dr. Yang, Jwing-Ming, he describes an artful, accurate path to the certain defeat of one's opponent. This is his description of the hand moving out to the first of the four corners.

> The right hand then changes into a palm, quickly threading forth beneath the left elbow, thrusting toward the opponent's rib cage and striking. There is no one who will not be dropped. In this form, the left and right hands thread reciprocally; suddenly hid-

den, suddenly appearing *(huyin huxian)* – unfathomable – *(zhuo mob u ding)* – attacking by seizing upon his emptiness. Thus, it is called Jade Maiden Threads Shuttle, in order to evoke the artfulness of the form.[6]

Narrative/Lived Experience
Weaving a Pattern...and Then Changing It

This sequence is sometimes called "Four Corners of the Universe," with the body and arm movements showing how we move out to each of the mythical "four corners." When I learned this sequence 24 years ago, the arms and hands took a more direct route from the body's center toward each corner. It took a while to remember the sequence... out to the left front, back to the center, out to the left rear, back to the center, out to the right rear, back to the center, out to the right front. The head, eyes, hips, shoulders, and foot travel out as one. The arms extend and the hands move out to shape the corner, then gently retract back in to hold the circle, rotate around to the next corner, and extend out again.

From time to time, a teacher can be inspired to change things up just a little – still honoring the lineage but adjusting the movements if it makes sense. A few years ago, my teacher Maedée Duprès hosted a retreat featuring an in-depth study of this sequence. We examined and learned a shift in the movements. This shift was more descriptive of the symbolism of "Fair Lady/Jade Maiden Works with Shuttles." The arms and hands still traveled out from the center, but they followed a weaving, spiraling motion out to each diagonal. This pattern meant that the outside arm took a more curved shape, while the outside shoulder extended slightly outward. This resembled the strategy to protect the vital organs, as suggested by Dr. Yang, Jwing-Ming.

The "Four Corners" order, and the location of each step, stayed the same. The torso moved out to each corner in the same manner. How-

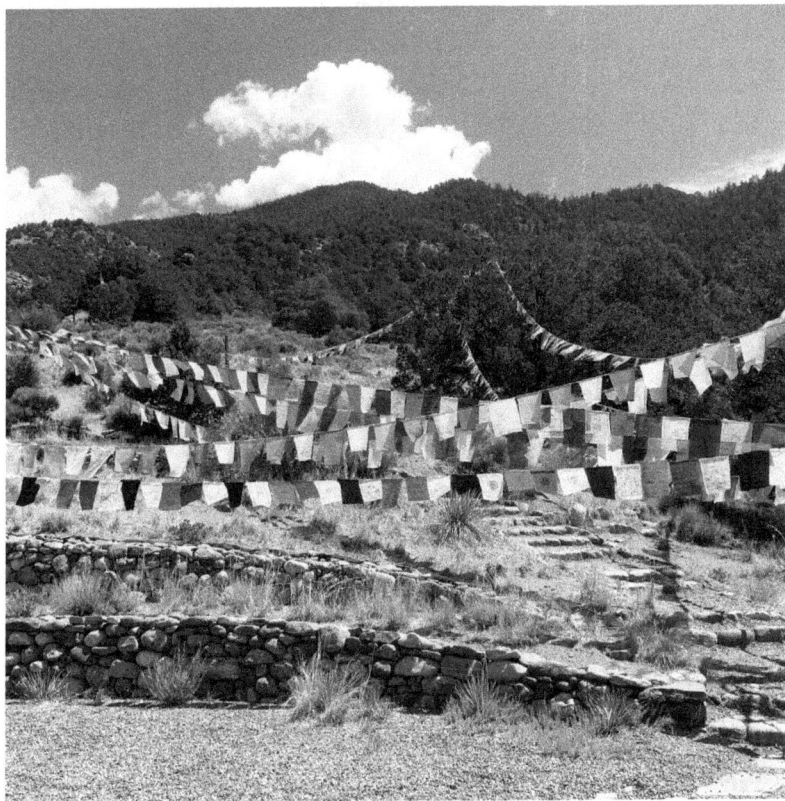

Patterns of color, form, and landscape suggest the Fair Lady weaving patterns at her loom.

ever, the new arm movements brought a fundamental change to the look and feel of the sequence.

For me, changing an established pattern is harder than learning something brand new, because I have to undo and redo the muscle memory. This takes time and patience, and the new Four Corners proved to be no exception to that rule. While I relearned the movements, my arms wouldn't cooperate. They either stuck to the old way or wandered around in vague and confusing arabesques. But eventually, the new movements took hold and became more clear, natural, and normal.

This process was made a little easier by remembering the wisdom of my teacher. She recognizes that the body and mind can put up a fierce resistance to change. When teaching revisions or making corrections, she points out that the difference will at first seem exaggerated and awkward. She encourages students to exaggerate the revision at first, a technique that adds clarity and gently deflects that instinctive resistance to change.

Making small changes in the form also reminds me that there's no absolute right or wrong way to practice tai chi ch'üan. Inflexibility does not serve me well, especially as I get older.

Where Am I?

The image of Kwan Yin is sometimes portrayed as a seated female figure with one foot extended out. This means that she is ready to rise from her seat and come quickly to the aid of anyone who is suffering.

I can count on her to show up when I need help, as she did one day in the post-surgery recovery room of a medical facility. I was in a chair next to my husband's bedside, waiting for him to open his eyes. I noticed the nurse was wearing a necklace in the image of Kwan Yin, and in that moment, a wave of recognition and relief washed over me. Kwan Yin's peaceful, smiling face and her mercy and compassion were a soothing balm for me, for the nurse, and for anyone in the room. She brought a little love and stability into the quicksand of anesthesia. For my husband, Kwan Yin was probably a vague image in a dense brain fog, but she was there.

The brain is not fond of uncertainty and the unknown. We're hardwired to avoid it. Neuroscientist Anne-Laure Le Cunff writes of a study from researchers at the University of Wisconsin–Madison, which shows how "uncertainty disrupts many of automatic cognitive processes that govern routine action. To ensure our survival, we become hypervigilant to potential threats. And this heightened state of worry creates conflict in the brain...When we feel uncertain about the future, doubt takes over our mind, making it difficult to think about anything else. Our mind is scattered and distracted. We feel like we're all over the place."[7]

The presence of Kwan Yin gently follows us as we flail around in the fog. I first met her in the Cleveland Museum of Art when I was 11 or 12 years old. At that time, my father worked at the museum and I often accompanied him to his office. Throughout the day, I'd wander through the galleries, often spending hours in one or two rooms. One day I found myself under the spell of Himalayan paintings from the 6th and 7th centuries. Green Tara, a manifestation of Kwan Yin, smiled out at me from her lotus seat. She was wearing an elaborate crown, striped pantaloons, and a whole lot of fancy jewelry. Her right foot gracefully extended from her bent knee. She was ready to come to the aid of the world.

Decades later, I ran across that same image on a bookmark, part of a display of impulse-buy items at the cash register in my favorite bookstore. As in the recovery room, I felt instant joyful recognition, like seeing a friend from long ago. I bought that bookmark, and Kwan Yin still smiles out at me from between the pages of a favorite book.

And most recently, Kwan Yin, or Green Tara, helped me to navigate a bout of anxiety and depression. I created a space inside my head for her image to dwell, breathing in and out with me. She sits there today, ready whenever I need her.

She also dwells in each of my t'ai chi ch'üan lessons. My teacher Maedée created a closing greeting called the Kwan Yin Aloha. We form a circle and perform a series of gestures indicating mercy and compassion for each other and for the universe. This seals the space in our minds, hearts, and spirits and offers respect and clarity to all the directions. Where am I? I am here. So are you. We added the name "aloha" at the suggestion of a student. Although it comes from a different culture, it is the right word for what we do.

Aloha is one of the most well-known Hawaiian words – both in the islands and around the world. As the song says, not only can aloha be used as a greeting, but also a farewell or good-bye. But there really is much more to this word…The term aloha derives from

Proto-Polynesia and dates back to the early 1800s. When broken down, the literal translation of the phrase translates to [Alo] meaning "presence" and [Hā] meaning "breath." Together the word aloha translates to "The presence of breath" or "breath of life."[8]

So we breathe in and out, into each of the four corners, and through the center and edges of the loom. Kwan Yin's strength and soothing presence reels us in from the unknown places.

Reflections of Mind, Body, and Intent

This sequence is among the most challenging with respect to finding one's orientation in space. The progression from one corner to the next can sometimes feel counterintuitive, out of order. On top of that, we are deprived of our visual connection when we turn to face the back

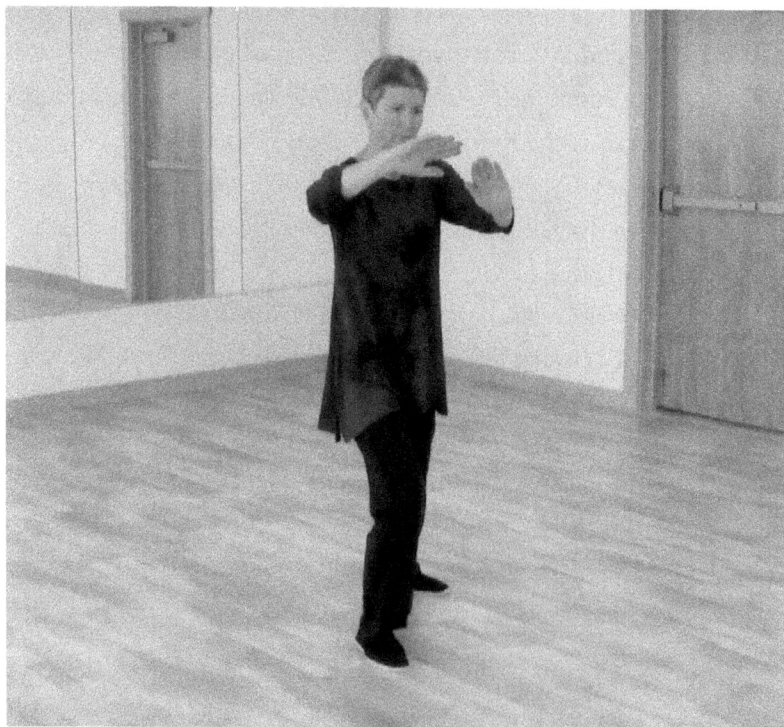

The hands do a weaving motion to imprint the shape of each corner.

and find ourselves completely on our own with no teacher to follow. Yikes…it must be the dark side of the moon!

Through practice, we gain confidence in the movement. We put our brains on the back burner, trust our muscle memory to guide us, and follow the dan tien, the geographical center of our body. We pass through the center of the loom, then gently weave the diagonal directions one by one, following the thread of the sequence. When this happens in a group, it's a magical experience. Each practitioner tunes in to someone else in the group but in a synchronized way, like a heartbeat. The movement aligns, and all the threads converge to follow the energy of the rotating center, gracefully, like ribbons around a maypole.

In Gerda Geddes's article "Turning Points" (Metamorphoses 1984), she reflects on the joy and mystery of seeking the four corners.

> There is a saying by Confucius: "If I give a student one corner of a subject and he does not find the other three corners for himself, I do not repeat my lesson. Master Choy [her t'ai chi teacher in the early 1950s] did just that for me. He gave me one corner, and looking for the other three to complete the picture has been an exciting search, like fitting together pieces in a jig-saw puzzle. Everything that I had learned before has been useful. Focusing towards the still point in the centre becomes synthesized with the ever widening circles of experience, so that in the end the centre and the circumference of the circle are experienced as one; or, as the mystics put it: "The centre of the circle is to be found everywhere."[9]

The author of *Tai Chi Chuan Classical Yang Style* describes Jade Maiden Threads Shuttle as intentional and artful. We too can be artful as we trace the sequence with the arms…precise, yet soft, cradling the chi within the shapes you form with each corner.

The feet and hands weave threads through a loom – following a pattern, back and forth, through the center, and to the outer edges. The shuttle carries the threads through the loom to create the pattern.

To travel to each of the four corners, the stepping-out foot traces a line of energy from the center of the loom, or the vertical axis. The line starts at the instep and travels out in accordance with the diagonal lunge. That same line is drawn after the torso rotates to the second, third, and fourth corners. Thus the foot and the torso delineate each corner of the square, inviting the whole body to stay deliberate, grounded, and focused toward each diagonal.

The arms move in spooling and unspooling spirals, showing more elements of the woven pattern, one color connecting to another and uniting in beauty and balance. The gentle reach of the shoulders follows this undulating pattern and follows the diagonal direction of the feet and hips.

The visual field widens as you gaze out to the distance through a little "window" formed by the index and middle fingers. With this gaze, the head on its long, supple neck tilts slightly to the right. The vision shifts to peripheral and the arms gather back in to the center as you Hold the Circle. This circle supports a strong and substantial vertical axis, smoothly turning as you travel from the center out to each subsequent corner.

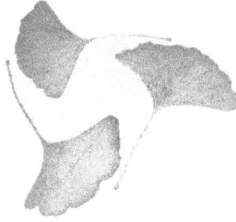

Chapter 11

Snake Creeps Down Into the Water

Symbolism, Tradition, and Background

This sequence is about transformation. The snake descends, sheds its skin, then rises from the water to become a bird.

Snakes shed their skins in order to grow. It's necessary – and astonishing – that this creature with no appendages can accomplish such a task. We too must sometimes transform, and that can be daunting. In *Looking for The Golden Needle,* Gerda Geddes notes that "An interesting aspect of the T'ai-chi Ch'üan is that when there is a movement of symbolic significance, like that of the snake, it is also very difficult to perform physically…"[1]

In *Tai Chi Chuan Classical Yang Style*, Dr. Yang, Jwing-Ming describes the wrapping and coiling imagery of a snake in search of prey.

The Chinese name of this form is "she shen xia shi." She means snake, shen means body. Xia means down or to lower, and shi means aspect or manner. The image is that of a snake wrapped around a branch, lowering its head as if about to attack. The name implies that you must first wrap, coil, stick and adhere with your opponent before you lower your body to attack. When a snake creeps down a branch, its head is lower than its body, searching the air to find and attack a target. (Dr. Yang, Jwing-Ming, 1999, page 298)[2]

During Snake Creeps Down, the extended left hand draws a full circle up, over to the right, down, left, and back up to be the snake's head emerging from the water. At that point the Golden Rooster Stands on One Leg.

The Chinese name of this form is "jin ji du li"....When a rooster stands on one leg, it is very stable and balanced. When you apply this form, you too must be balanced and stable. (Dr. Yang, Jwing-Ming, 1999, page 299)[3]

How do we maintain balance and stability while the body travels through space, then pivots and rises up from bent knees to stand on one leg? By staying in the center of the circle.

The founder of Yang style t'ai chi, Yang Luchan, was described as small and slight of build, but able to throw adversaries twice his size. He is said to have reacted to any stimulus as if he were a solid, rotating sphere. In *The Dao of Taijuquan*, the author states:

The purpose of taijiquan is to train to…become like a dynamic…rotating sphere which, for the martial arts, is the most balanced and beautiful of all shapes. Note that the center of gravity and the point of support are always aligned with the line of the center of gravity in every possible orientation of the sphere…and hence, no instability can be induced.[4]

Thus, if our *dan tien* is in line with the weight and the vertical axis, our snake smoothly descends, sheds, and rises. The line of energy travels through the sequence.

T'ai Chi Classics makes reference to this principle in Master Wu Yu-Hsiang's treatise.

Transfer of power comes from the spine. Change of position follows the movement of your body.

The transfer of power roots at the foot, travels through the leg, and is controlled by the waist. The waist serves the same function as the transmission in an automobile: it distributes the amount and direction of your power. After long periods of practice and success in T'ai Chi stance and rooting techniques, the transfer of power will be directly from the waist, following the spine up to the shoulder, and eventually reaching the fingertips. Control of the process of transferring power is therefore located in and mainly depends on your spinal column.[5]

If the body is stable and rooted throughout this sequence, we have some space to reflect on change. In *The Dao of Taijiquan*, Jou, Tsung Hwa notes:

The concept of change as expressed in the *Yijing* plays a very important role in taijiquan's system. The *Yijing* states that everything changes or develops through certain cycles. Nothing is constant but change itself…The practical applications of this principle in taijiquan are endless.[6]

He then goes on to describe several points about the nature of change, including:

In the practice of taijiquan, the concept of change is integrated as the system of study…For instance, in the posture Snake Creeps Down you know the principles which must not be violated: feet flat on the floor, body upright, constant height, etc…The execution of this posture is up to you as long as you maintain the unchanging points, and this fact allows the posture to change and develop.[7]

Gerda Geddes suggests that the t'ai chi itself shows us the way through transformation of the whole self.

> …these succeeding stages of awakening in the T'ai-chi Ch'üan have to be enacted by the body. It is as if the T'ai-chi Ch'üan says "Always remember that as long as you are in this life you must live through the wholeness of yourself, not just the body in one place and the spirit in another."[8]

Narrative/Lived Experience

Being in the "Uh-Oh" Moment

The first sequence of Snake Creeps Down Into the Water occurs about two-thirds of the way through the form, and it is repeated again near the end. In Looking for The Golden Needle, Geddes's interpretation emphasizes transformation, enacted by the body in a profound test of strength, flexibility, and endurance.

Let's return to the idea of shedding. What is being shed might resist being let go of, whether it's the snake's skin or an object or idea we no longer need. There are several stages: recognition, preparation, the process of shedding, and the emergence as a transformed being. All require a lot of energy and concentration. And if there's not enough juice left at the very end, saved for the new snake to emerge out of the water, that can mean big trouble.

One of my lived experiences related to Snake Creeps Down Into the Water came during a time when my life was transforming. I learned the hard way (as usual) how to assess my limitations and allocate my energy.

This lesson came in an unexpected place: Whole Foods, where I'd stopped after a physical therapy appointment. The therapist had recommended a stability ball to help me build balance and strength following a life-threatening infection, spinal surgery, and eight days in the hospital. I was weak and fragile…as puny as I'd ever been. I located the supply of stability balls on a lower shelf.

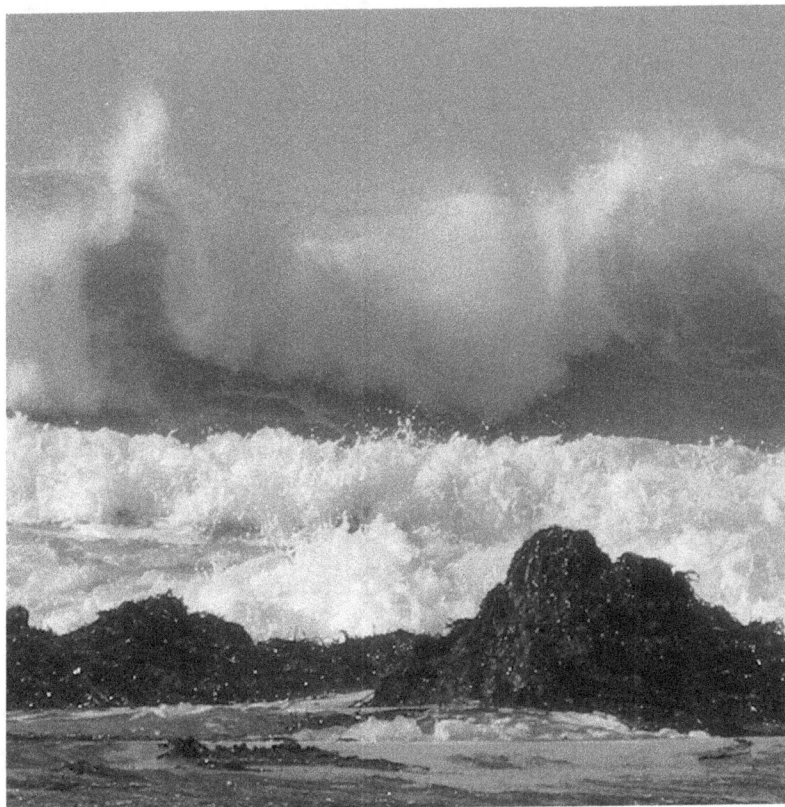

We can tap into the powerful, buoyant energy of water during Snake Creeps Down.

I was still in the early stages of healing, so bending over to reach to the floor wasn't yet an option. Heaven forbid I should ask for help, so…t'ai chi to the rescue! I felt that I had the perfect solution to the problem. So I set my feet, opened my knees and lowered myself in the Snake Creeps Down position so I could reach the merchandise. So far, so good, but…when I started the ascent…oops. My leg strength, like the rest of me, was seriously diminished.

The puny self that I was in that moment was very far from the stronger self of a few months earlier. That meant I was stuck at the bottom of the ocean. If I wanted to get up off the floor and take that ball home, I'd need to make myself more buoyant. My legs weren't strong enough to help me muscle through this problem. I carefully shifted my weight back onto both heels and brought my feet into parallel. From there I managed to use willpower and the nearby shelves to ratchet myself up to vertical, pay for the ball, and head home for a nap.

We're often encouraged to "live in the moment" and learn from the experience. In that moment – not one of my finest – I got a lesson in letting go of stuff I didn't need to carry: pride and an inaccurate estimate of my own strength. Accepting and trusting my vulnerable, transforming self was necessary, just like it's necessary for the snake to shed its old skin.

Six months went by before I felt like "myself" once more. I had a long and painful road ahead, with no assurance that I would fully recover. But by leaving that skin behind, at least I was lighter to take my first steps in those weird and scary present moments.

The Buoyancy of Community

During that long winter of 2006, my path of recovery from back surgery was transformed and supported by my community of practitioners. On January 6, the day of my surgery, four of my t'ai chi colleagues were gathered a few miles away with our teacher Maedée Duprès, who was teaching the second of four weekend intensives. These three-day programs were components of a year-long t'ai chi ch'üan teacher certification program I'd embarked on a couple of months earlier. Each of these intensives included a research topic presented by a student, and on January 6, that student was Ed Berg.

Ed had studied with Maedée for a number of years. He was a delightful mix of practicality, energy, curiosity, and humor. He was a skillful and dedicated practitioner who shunned the uber-mystical cachet that's sometimes attached to t'ai chi. "It ain't precious," he would say with a grin and a twinkle in his eye.

Ed had a successful career in petroleum geophysics, and a poet's heart inspired by his love of nature. This shone out in his presentation, which began with a section "What Tai Chi Means to Me."

The great and life-long value of Tai Chi is that it is an exercise that is rooted in and lives within both the physical and spiritual dimensions we each have…It is something real that happens within your body and in your mind or spirit, not outside of you. What it means will be different for each one of you, and it will constantly change from this moment onward. Let me try to illustrate a little of what it has come to mean to me:

When I was a boy, my grandfather lived on an inlet
off a bay in the north.
He had a handmade wooden skiff with a five-horse outboard motor,
And he would take me fishing in it when we visited him.
We'd putter slowly past the neighbors' docks
and safely moored boats
Until we came to where the familiar banks fell away,
And the far shore went out and out,
Until it disappeared in the skyline haze.
Then Gramps would ease the throttle open and the little boat
would pick up speed,
Lifting on the broad-backed swells that came in
from long and far away,
Where the wind had room to work,
and the bottom went down deep.
The first time it happened, I gripped the gunwales
in an instant of panic,
At the new and unbalancing motion,
but soon relaxed into the competence
Of the old man and the willing little boat,
and rode easy on the water.
Over and again, long after those times slipped past
on the curling wake of the little boat,
At moments when I first grasp some new idea,
Or when a song quickens something true deep within,

That lifting, speeding moment in the boat on the open water
comes back to visit,
And I am reminded that the best things we can do,
or understand, or give away,
Are empowered by a swelling immensity
that arises from some great depth below us,
And all we can do is steer with the best skill we have,
Point the bow into the wind, and let the waters carry us on our way.

…The image of water is central to the movement and thought of Tai Chi. The idea, or actually the whole philosophy, is called in Chinese "wu wei," and it translates literally as "doing without doing," but what it means is more like, "acting with the least possible force.[9]

Ed expressed his own version of the allegorical journey through water, then offered an invitation. "I want you too, to be lifted on the swells that arise in your own depths, and be carried in delight on your way."[10]

In this manner, our metaphorical Snake sheds its skin to be lightened for its transformation, rises out of the depths, and becomes the Golden Bird. Joyful momentum is what's needed to complete this movement as a strong, stable, square, golden creature with wings.

A couple of weeks after coming home from the hospital, I found myself wanting nothing more than to return to the teacher certification group and try to finish up the program. It was a shaky proposition but thanks to my teacher and colleagues, I did it. Ed's written words encouraged me: "Tai Chi is a way of thinking and moving that will help you to walk, spiritually and physically, with grace and strength and purpose, on your lifelong pathway."[11]

Ed and his wife Paula moved to Salida in 2005, and I saw him occasionally in the years that followed. He had a wonderful life there and passed away peacefully in his sleep on October 17, 2022. His obituary in the *Salida Mountain Mail* reads in part, "Family and friends said he was more than a husband, father and friend – he was intensely curious, a Renaissance man, a craftsman, philosopher, artist and athlete."[12]

His words hold meaning, strength, and buoyancy of body, mind, spirit. The buoyancy is what sweeps us onward and upward, with courage and perseverance. Halfway around the Taoist yin-yang circle, we encounter the same principle, mirrored. As we kick out, we gain strength and stability from the counterbalance…groundedness. As we creep down like snakes to the bottom of the sea, we gain momentum from the counterbalance…buoyancy.

Reflections of Mind, Body, and Intent

The movement of Snake Creeps Down Into The Water asks a lot of the body. But when the moving parts collaborate, the Snake feels magical. It's full of nuance: just enough muscle but not too much. Smooth rotation and open joints follow a complete circle with no sticky spots or compression. The intent of momentum is essential.

The snake is one of two main characters in the apocryphal story about the founder of tai chi, Chang San-Feng (1279-1368 AD). According to legend, Chang San-Feng observed a fight between a crane and a snake. The crane stabbed with its beak, but the snake twisted out of reach. This sparked Chang San-Feng's study of other movements in nature and the basis for many fundamental ideas: yin and yang, yielding in the face of strength, and moving in a manner that keeps effort to a minimum.

The snake's graceful movements have inspired writers and thinkers everywhere. Emily Dickinson's poem "A narrow Fellow in the Grass" describes "A Whip-Lash unbraiding in the sun."[13] This makes me think of the Single Whip unbraiding to become a snake, then a golden bird.

Rudyard Kipling's python Kaa in *The Jungle Book* "seemed to pour his way across the ground."[14] Our snake can gently but powerfully pour, a force of nature navigating the unfamiliar braidings and unbraidings of our bodies, minds, and lives.

The sense of chi flowing through the vertical axis, or plumb line, supports a snake that navigates the challenge of shedding its skin to rise

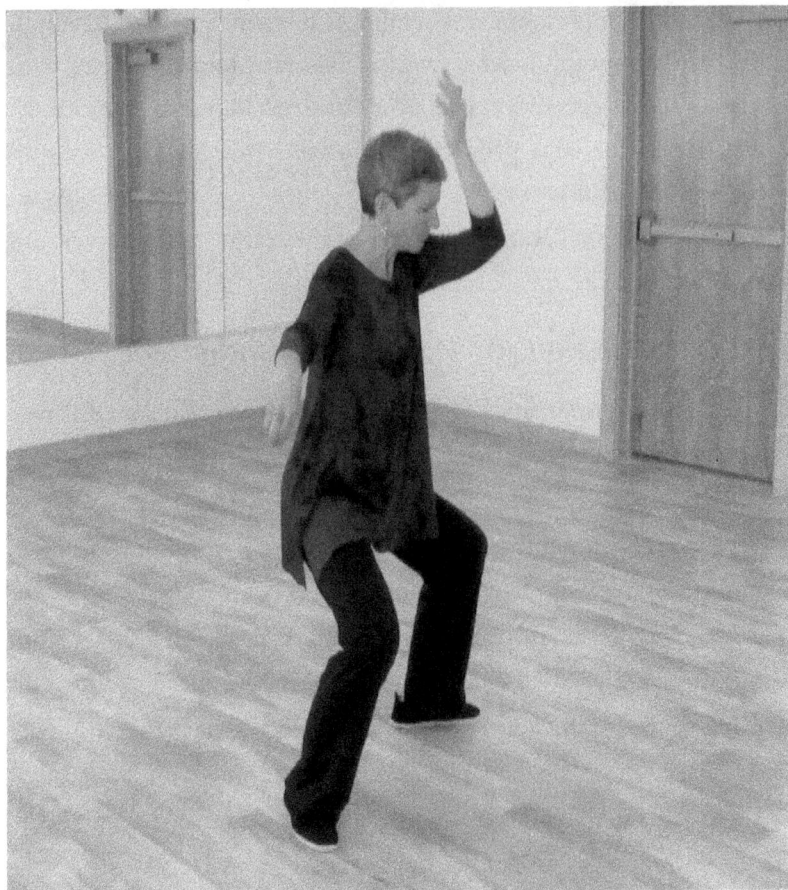

The Snake sheds its skin, transforming to become as light and strong as a Golden Bird.

out of the water and transform into a bird. If the limbs are synchronized with the vertical axis, they add further support and encouragement to all the movements of the vertical axis: shifting right, sinking downward, gliding to the left, and then rising up.

As you sink, think of the knees and legs as powerful hydraulic mechanisms. They are most efficient when they take the path of least resistance, acting with steady strength and no obstacles to the flow. As the knees bend, carefully fine-tune the alignment over the ankles and feet. The little turn-out on the right foot widens the stance to help keep the knees and hips open – like a big yawn.

Visualize the spine as a straight but supple stem that tilts just a little bit forward, so as to relieve pressure on the hips and legs. As you lower yourself down to the bottom of the sea, imagine that the water you're in supports that descent. At the lowest point, the right foot pivots and the right knee rotates inward. This is when the snake sheds its skin, bringing a sense of lightness as the weight shifts to the left leg. Inhale to move upward and forward, as if you are floating up while riding an ocean current. A gentle boost with the back leg gives just enough help.

As the snake creeps down, the arm movements support and clarify the movements of the legs and torso as they tell the story of transformation. They draw the spacious boundaries of the energy sphere: up over the head, out to the side, downward, and up out of the water as the snake sheds its skin. The left hand shows the snake coming out of the water, fingers tilting upward and forward, like the head of a little sea-creature taking a breath of air. The right hand is the Golden Bird's stately and powerful wing, forming a right angle as the bird squares up to stand on the left leg. In the final movement of this sequence, the Golden Bird shows its strength and symmetry as the left leg rises up and forward to rest, tall and triumphant, on the right leg.

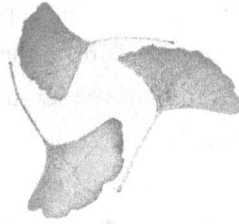

Chapter 12

High Pat on the Horse

Symbolism, Tradition, and Background

T'ai chi ch'üan sequence names can invite the body to respond instinctively and naturally to a posture or phrase. Open the Bird's Wing is a good example. When we say or think of the name, perhaps that evokes the idea of opening our own wing. Then, the body responds to the cue and often, the movement feels and looks deeply beautiful.

But High Pat on the Horse...what message does that send to the body? In *The Essence and Applications of Taijiquan*, Yang Chengfu describes how to do the movement and offers some background on its intention and meaning.

Loosen the waist and contain the chest...the eyes look forward. The slight raising of the spine and back has the intention both of stretching and drawing upward, and advancing forward *(tan ba qian jin)*.

Translator's Comments: Conventionally translated "High Pat on the Horse," the Chinese name…calls upon imagery that may reflect special familiarity with matters equestrian. The verb *tan* means "to test, to put out a feeler, to explore, spy, scout," as well as the physical motion of "stretching forth." All of these connections apply in the posture, which requires a rising up and a stretching forth. There is, incidentally, a compound, *tanma*, which means a mounted scout. Xu Yusheng evokes this in his explanation of the form name: "The body towers upward, reaching outward to the front, rather like the appearance of being mounted on a horse, with the body reaching forward."[1]

For this same sequence, Dr. Yang, Jwing-Ming also refers to the intent of searching upward and outward. But he names it Stand High to Search Out the Horse. "The Chinese name of this form is 'gao tan ma.' Gao means high, tan means to try or search out, and ma means horse. When you search for your horse in the field, you must use your hands to shade your eyes from the sun in order to see far and clear." (Dr. Yang, Jwing-Ming, 1999, page 248)[2]

This sequence invites a sense of reaching outward, scouting, then landing gently. The hands float past each other as they reach out to the left diagonal. High Pat on the Horse is first performed as the lead-in to the kicking section and again near the end of Part Three.

In both instances, the arms reach toward to the left diagonal, the hands pass each other, and the body roots itself on the diagonal. However, there's a small yet significant difference in the hand position for the second instance that opened the door for Gerda Geddes's reflection on crossed hands and divergent energy.

Since I moved up to Scotland four years ago, the two last sequences of the Tai Chi Chuan have become very clear, starting with Crossing the Arms [the ending position of High Pat on the Horse]. One force moving up, the other force moving down, Yang floating up and away, Yin staying down rooted to the earth. This movement became associated with the death of my husband. I was devastated. Grief completely took over my life, I was reaching the bottom. It took about a year until one day I woke up feeling light and cheerful and thinking, life must go on. I was able to let David go, to set him free and thereby also freeing myself, preparing for the last sequence.[3]

This passage reminds me of the difficulty of "going on." Nothing moves on until there is some sort of release. Sometimes this feels like a tight knot that's impossible to untangle. Suppose it's a knot in a necklace with a very fine chain. And suppose you chose that necklace to wear to work, and you're late because you tried, wasting even more time, to undo the knot – without success. Later, when you have time, you lay the chain down on a smooth, flat surface and gently shake it around to give the knot some space. Then the tight loops can be wiggled loose so as to gently tease the knot open.

In the same manner, I can also encourage flow and spaciousness in my t'ai chi ch'üan practice if I am patient and relaxed.

Relaxing is fundamental to the practice, and easier said than done. As Cheng Man-ch'ing, a student of Yang Chengfu, wrote in Master Cheng's Thirteen Chapters on T'ai Chi Ch'üan:

Every day Master Yang repeated at least ten times: "Relax! Relax! Be calm. Release the whole body." Otherwise he would say, "You're not relaxed! You're not relaxed! Not being relaxed means that you are in a position to receive a beating." Note: The one word "relax" is the most difficult to achieve. If one can truly be calm, then all the rest comes naturally.[4]

The term sung appears in many resources as a central principle in the movement. In The Essence of T'ai Chi Ch'uan, the third of Yang Chengfu's 10 points states:

Sung (relax) the waist. The waist is the commander of the whole body. If you can sung the waist, then the two legs will have power and the lower part will be firm and stable.[5]

Sung implies a sort of dynamic relaxation. Think of the supple movement of the waist in a sequence like Waving Arms Like Clouds. That is sung. Relaxed yet lively.

Number 5 of Yang Chengfu's 10 points addresses another facet of relaxing.

Sink the shoulders and elbows. The shoulders should be completely relaxed and open. If you cannot relax and sink, the two shoulders will be "uptight." The *chi* (breath) will follow them up and the whole body cannot get power.[6]

To relax and sink, again we maintain the liveliness and flow, so as not to collapse and compress the spine. Sink, but stay upright...it's a delicate balance, almost contradictory. It makes sense if we keep our energy connection to the yang, the upward intent. Then the sinking and relaxing has the effect of bringing openness and spaciousness to the spine and all the other joints from head to toe.

Narrative/Lived Experience

When we reach the sequences of High Pat on the Horse to the Halfway Down Punch, we're almost 90% of the way through the form. We've practiced many sequences many times, and they are becoming familiar to our minds and established in our muscle memory. In this sequence, we use our experience and skill to execute a big rotation in the hip joints, call on single-leg strength, and carefully square up and relax the body for one last kick.

When teaching this sequence, I stress the need to be relaxed and patient with the body as it makes its way around the circle to prepare for the kick. It's precarious, and premature, to execute a kick while the body is still making its way around from the High Pat, so we need time for a proper set-up. And since we're close to the end, we're tired, so it can be a challenge to move slowly. But if we do, we are rewarded with a stable and spacious platform, allowing the chi to gather and flow. Then we can send out the kick, smoothly delivering power out through the foot.

At this point in the form, keeping an eye on our energy reserves is important. "Finish strong" is an endurance-sport truism, but it is useful and relevant to many other activities.

I learned the value of "finishing strong" through experience. And as is so often the case for me, I learned by first ignoring, then applying, a wise person's advice.

In 2004, I took part in Ride the Rockies, a long-distance cycling event held annually in Colorado. Part of my preparation was taking a class in basic bike repair and maintenance. The instructor, who'd ridden the event a number of times, taught us the mechanical details and also gave us a few tips on the ride itself. For the big, multiple-mile climbs that would greet us every day of the six-day ride, she said, "Make sure you have a couple of gears left in reserve when you reach the top." Save some juice and finish strong, in other words.

On the first day of Ride the Rockies, I failed the first of many "finish strong" tests that came my way during the event. That day's route took us a few miles north out of our starting point in Boulder, then west on Lefthand Canyon Drive. The road climbed more and more steeply before tilting up in a 10% grade just below the little town of Ward.

I'd prepared diligently for several months, gradually building miles per week, adding weekend rides of 50-60 miles, and logging a few big, long climbs in the mountains. Nonetheless, I was a little nervous on this first day.

I'd read about the "personality" of this event. The 2,000+ participants ranged from serious ultra-endurance athletes to gung-ho middle schoolers to aging oddballs. I veered more toward the last category. I was riding my trusty mountain bike with straight handlebars instead of

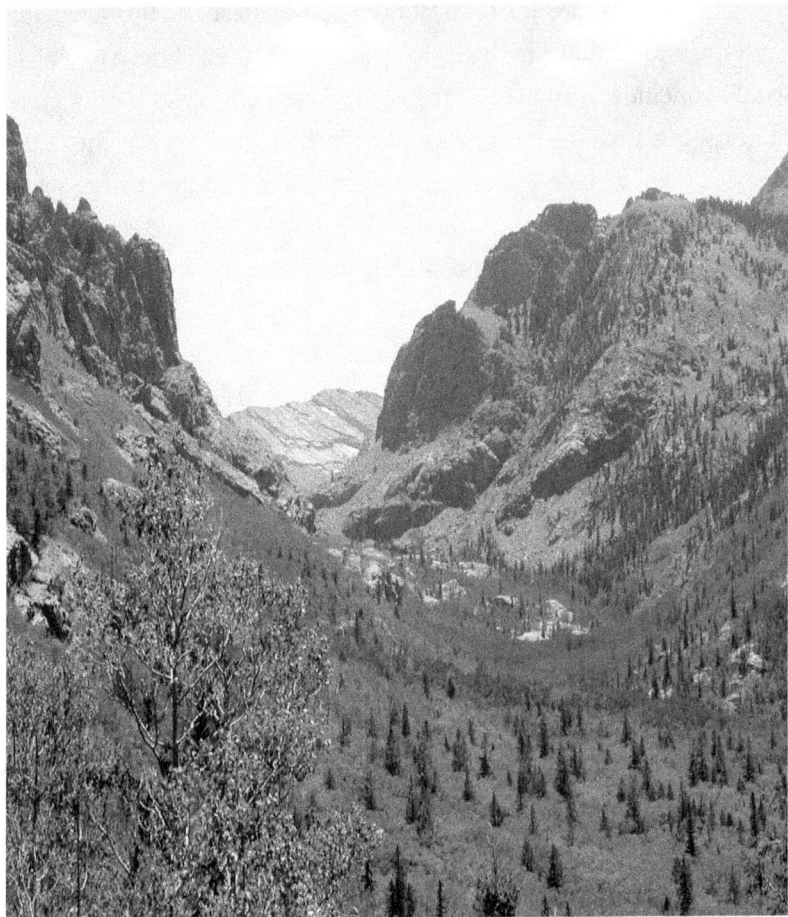

On this hike, the top kept getting farther away...but patience paid off.

a lean, fast, greyhound-like road bike. I had made only a small conces-sion for Ride the Rockies by switching out my knobby mountain-bike tires for more road-friendly smooth ones.

As was my custom, I carried a small backpack containing water and a few items of clothing. I was too cheap to buy one of those fan-cy, multi-pocketed bicycle shirts to store gear for the day. As I ped-aled northwest on Highway 36, my outfit and my ride prompted some snickers and snide comments from a swiftly passing herd of riders. 'I'll see you in Estes Park,' I muttered to myself.

A couple of hours later, we labored up the dreaded 10% grade toward the intersection with highway 7 and the final leg of the day, which would conclude in an overnight stop in Estes Park. I was running out of gears, but I was still pedaling and I still had some juice in the tank. But just then, I made a classic mistake: I glanced up the road to see if I could spot the top. That little shift in attention allowed the force of gravity to gain the upper hand, and in an instant I was moving almost too slowly to stay upright.

But the top was only a couple of switchbacks away...and more importantly, I saw an unlikely yet profoundly motivating force – a rider who appeared to be in his 70s, wearing a full tuxedo and a top hat, happily and easily pedaling upward on the switchback right above me. I thought, 'Well damn, if he can do it, I can, too.' I gritted my teeth and willed myself upward on nonexistent muscle power. It was ego that got me to the top, but extra juice would have helped.

That wasn't the only test of my endurance that day. After the big hill and Tuxedo Man came a rolling 15-mile stretch, followed by a long descent into Estes Park. Just as we started down the hill, at an altitude of about 9,000 feet, a thunderstorm hit. This triggered another endurance-event coping strategy – motivating myself with the fear of not arriving at the end of the day in a vertical and conscious state.

Fear energy is very strong, but it needs a firm hand on the reins. The road was slippery, the rain was pelting down, and my brakes were wet. At that point I was glad to have my relatively hefty tires. I thought of their width and breadth as I navigated the winding road downward. Finally, the grade grew more level and the outskirts of Estes Park beckoned. I joined a miserable group huddling under the eaves of a 7-Eleven and got my wits together.

On the final quarter-mile into town the fear slowly dissolved out of me and with it, the rest of the energy "juice" I had regained on the level stretch after Tuxedo Man Hill. I met up with my son and we headed to our hotel. It rained all night, and as I warmed up under a warm, dry blanket, I thought of a classic bumper sticker: Nature bats last.

Looking out at the streetlights reflecting on the wet pavement the next morning, I reminded myself of my goal for Ride the Rockies: Prepare enough to have fun. I had built up an adequate supply of physical endurance to support that goal, but on that first day, I forgot about patience, acceptance, and extra juice. Perhaps the sequences of High Pat on the Horse and Halfway Down Punch ask for those same qualities, when we are close enough to taste the finish line but still a little bit out of reach.

Reflections of Mind, Body, and Intent

These sequences invite us to work through a challenge by tapping into what has been learned, taking the path of least resistance, and patiently adjusting in the moment. Then we open up, relax, and let go of the burden of doing it "right." We can enjoy a fluid and joyful movement, in the moment, as we travel to the next sequence.

Stephen T. Asma, a philosophy professor and musician, reflected on the magic and vulnerability of being "in the now." His article about musical improvisation, "Was Bo Diddley a Buddha?" appeared in the *New York Times* in 2017.

We relax and open up when we invite a sense of curiosity and "come what may" to the natural, easeful movement of t'ai chi ch'üan. Asma describes the idea.

"Wu-Wei" is a Chinese word that is often translated as "non-action" but more accurately means "natural action," or action in accordance with nature. The idea, dominant in Taoism and Zen, is that one should try to find the natural way of doing something and then simulate, or align oneself to it, as opposed to forcing it... Finding this natural way is not effortless, but requires great practice. Once it has been mastered, however, it is possible to find a unique presence of mind in these activities...The improvisational mind is typically an underappreciated source of wisdom.[7]

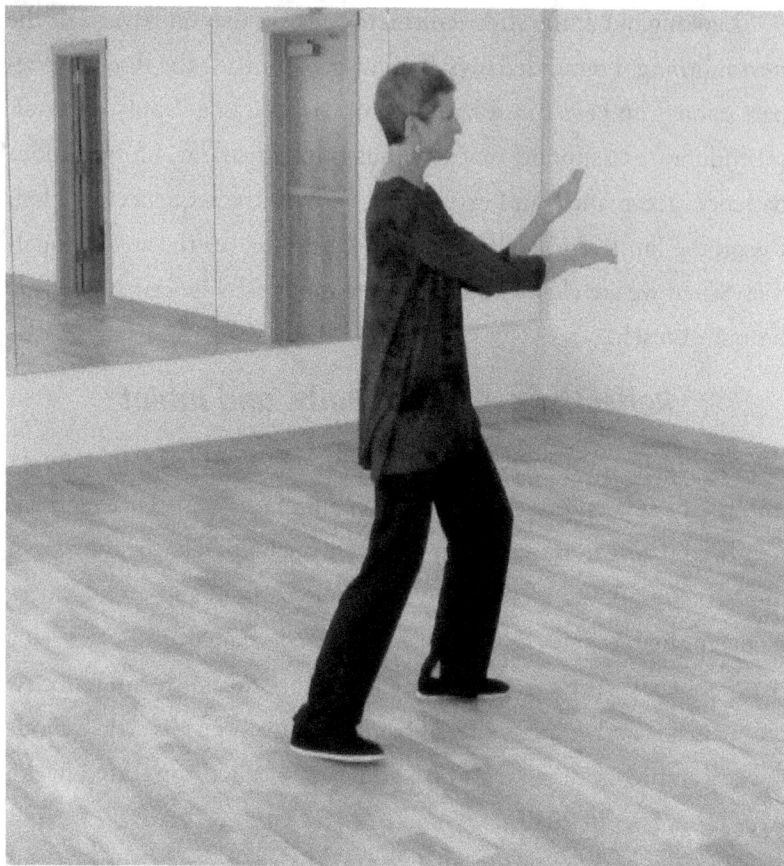

The crossed-hand energy changes as the body changes direction.

In these sequences we use our knowledge and experience to explore movements – unspooling the body from west to east, undoing the knots of crossed energy, then directing energy smoothly and powerfully outward – all with patience and intent toward a stable, relaxed self.

As discussed earlier in this chapter, there is a small but significant change in the second occurrence of High Pat on the Horse. At the end of the first occurrence of this phrase, wrists are crossed and both palms face you. In the second High Pat, the wrists are crossed but the right palm faces downward and the left upward. The backs of the hands face each other and thus the energy has a dissonant or "crossed" feel.

This is resolved as the body turns to prepare for the kick and Halfway Down Punch.

As the torso and legs travel around the half-circle, the hands stay in their crossed position until the body nears the end of the turn. The right arm rotates and the palm turns to face inward. This can call up the image of undoing a knot in a necklace. If the knot is stubborn, give the tangled part some space by setting it on a tabletop and gently jiggling it. Notice how this idea helps the body to manage this twisty sequence. Allow the hips to negotiate the turn in manageable increments so that you arrive at the end of the half-turn with hip joints open, wide, and ready to unspool into the kick. It's the very last kick, so let the empty leg move smoothly and easily away from the hip. Minimize the effort and notice how the leg can loosely ride the air currents. The wide, soft shoulders also feel easy and open. The hands unfurl and mirror the heel-ball-toe journey of the kicking foot.

Ask the muscle memory to kick in for the twisted step, slowly rotating to prepare for the Halfway Down Punch. At the same time, gently remind the body of the slight variances of this position: Left fingers tilt up as if holding a fan, spine tilts slightly forward for a slightly lower punch. Hands sketch the same shape of the moving spoke and the quiet hub of your turning "wheel."

As the right fist releases, imagine the intricate and well-designed interior of a clock, gears meshing smoothly to complete the eighth-turn and finish the sequence in the Ward Off position.

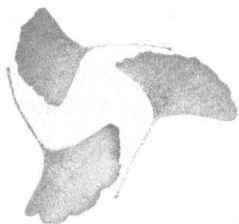

Chapter 13

Riding the Crane to the Seven Stars, Shoot Out the Arrow

Symbolism, Tradition, and Background

The finishing movements of the t'ai chi ch'üan are so rich in symbolism and meaning. We Ride the Crane to the Seven Stars, then gently release the soul to its journey outward. Then the body returns to tranquil stability, represented by one more Twisted Step and Punch, and one last Carry Tiger to the Mountain. We finish where we started – full circle.

This movement group, sometimes called the Grand Terminus, marks the end of our allegorical journey – a life well-lived. With celebration, solemnity, and focus, we bring our training and experience to bear as we move through the final stages of life.

Riding the Crane to the Seven Stars refers to the Big Dipper constellation. As with many other sequences, the symbolism of the name has more than one interpretation. Regardless of how it connects to a physical movement, it evokes the Seven Stars, twinkling in the far reaches of the night sky.

Dr Yang, Jwing-Ming links the constellation to body position. As he writes in *Tai Chi Chuan Classical Yang Style* (in which the sequence is titled Step Forward to the Seven Stars):

> The Chinese name of this form is "shang bu qi xing." Shang bu means step forward, and qi xing means seven stars. In China, the seven stars refer to the seven stars of the big dipper. In this form your body resembles the constellation, with your front leg the handle and your body and arms the bowl. (Dr. Yang, Jwing-Ming, 1999, page 328)[1]

He also offers a fighting context for the movements of the body in this sequence.

> Chinese people believe that the arrangement of the seven stars hides many fighting strategies. For example, qi xing zhen, which means seven star tactics, refers to ways of positioning and moving troops in battle. Qi xing bu means seven star steps and refers to ways of stepping and moving in combat. Qi xing is also used to refer to the cavities located on the chest. In this form you step forward to form the qi xing form and strike your opponent's qi xing area. (Dr. Yang, Jwing-Ming, 1999, page 328)[2]

Then we Step Back and Ride the Tiger, or "step back to pass over the tiger." (Dr. Yang, Jwing-Ming, 1999, page 329)[3] This takes bravery, stability, and finesse.

> The tiger is a very powerful and violent animal. If you desire to ride one, you had better hold on to the hair on his back tightly, otherwise you will fall and become his victim. If you want to pass over a sleeping tiger, you must also be careful not to touch the tiger and wake him. Generally speaking, this form implies that your

hands hold onto the opponent, and your steps should be careful to set up the most advantageous position for yourself. (Dr. Yang, Jwing-Ming, 1999, page 329)[4]

He offers further analysis. "You must…first increase your stability by sitting back as if you were riding a tiger: firm and stable." (Dr. Yang, Jwing-Ming, 1999, page 329)[5]

From there, the intent shifts as we Pick up the Lotus Flower. "The feel …is like a lotus leaf on a long stem, swinging from side to side in the wind. (Dr. Yang, Jwing-Ming, 1999, page 330)[6]

Dr. Yang, Jwing-Ming's description of a long stem swinging comes alive in a video clip of Gerda Geddes doing t'ai chi ch'üan in the City Park in Bergen, Norway. In "The Magic Bird Spreads its Wings," a program that aired on Norwegian TV in 1989, we see a dynamic, agile lady performing the t'ai chi ch'üan in a public park. As park visitors pass by, some stop and watch curiously. When she "picks up the lotus flower," her right leg slowly and rhythmically swings, like a long, powerful stem infused with pure natural grace and the fluid strength of chi.

I've often shown this video clip to students to share my sense of wonder, inspiration, and delight. She makes it look so easy! Infused throughout the video is her cheery, unflappable demeanor. Her narrated words, as well as her facial expression, remind the audience to not take themselves too seriously and to cherish a sense of play, even in life's biggest moments.

In *Looking for The Golden Needle,* Ms. Geddes offers her insight on the Grand Terminus.

Finally, we come to the last sequence where there is a repetition of Snake Creeps Down Into the Water, but this time the snake emerges out of the water having been transformed into a movement called **Reaching for the Seven Stars.** These are the stars of the Great Dipper. The aim of the Taoist sage was to ride on the back of a crane up to the seven stars when it was time for him to depart from this life. In the next movement you prepare yourself to **Ride the Tiger.** When you Ride the Tiger, it means that you are in full control of your energy and your Ch'i. It was thought that a sage could decide on the moment of his departure when he had mastered the art of riding the tiger. Next you **Pick Up the Lotus Flower With the Leg.** The lotus is the Golden Flower of Taoism, the crystalization of the experience of light. The lotus also represents everything that is beautiful, so before you depart from this world, you pick up the lotus as if to say "Thank you for everything that was beautiful in this life."[7]

When we Ride the Crane to the Seven Stars, we launch the soul on its journey – and the lighter it is, the better. Thus, in Part Three, we twice perform Snake Creeps Down Into the Water. Each time, the snake sheds its skin at the bottom of the sea, so as to become more buoyant for the transformative journey to the seven stars.

The t'ai chi ch'üan invites us to tell a transformation story with our bodies. For that reason, I often draw on thoughts and words from outside the practice and its traditions. Then, my mind and body form a partnership, bringing me closer to the idea of "moving meditation."

One of my favorite experiences of this partnership came from a passage in N. Scott Momaday's *Earth Keeper: Reflections on the American Land.* I was so inspired by it that I recently read it to a group of students during a lesson on Riding the Crane to the Seven Stars.

In one particular passage, Momaday speaks with power and eloquence of that same journey, and how it is a bridge that connects us to the stars and all of the natural world. The moment of death is a significant transition and a release. The poem speaks of traveling to a place far away, with joy and anticipation, toward the stars in distant camps.

Momaday's writing goes right to my heart and soul. The words paint a portrait of the human experience, which we also enact in the t'ai chi ch'üan. When it's ready, the spirit takes wing on the breeze, effortlessly spiraling off toward the seven stars like the buoyant feathers of a milkweed seed.

Narrative/Lived Experience

We Ride the Cranes

I taught t'ai chi ch'üan on Tuesdays and Thursdays at the Schless-man YMCA in Denver, Colorado for about eight years. Although the class format was drop-in and for all levels, about a third of the group consisted of a strong community of "regulars." With dedication and perseverance, they gradually learned the Yang style long form over a period of several years.

As they slowly learned the form, I slowly became acquainted with regulars and not-so-regulars; answering questions, chatting about fine points of the form, and catching up before and after class about recent vacations, life changes, and weather.

Speaking of weather, not once in those eight years was I "stood up" on the wintry mornings when I'd slog through snow, ice, and chill, making my way to the Y with a sense of futility. Who in their right mind would show up on a day like this? In the studio, I'd shake off the snow, change my shoes, and in would stroll the intrepid Catherine, a Minnesota native who had a "so what" attitude toward the worst that winter could dole out. Then, almost always, four or five others would trickle in. I am forever grateful for their dedication.

The regulars all had their favorite spots in the studio. Catherine's was in the middle of the back row. I encouraged students to switch spots occasionally so they could pick up on different details of the move-ments. Nonetheless, seeing them in their chosen spaces felt comfort-able, like a family gathering around the dinner table.

Another regular attendee was Phoebe, a retired educator whose presence inspired and energized me. Her clear, insightful questions supported everyone in the group – a valuable gift, as many students, especially new ones, tended to be reticent about speaking up in a group setting. From her preferred spot, up front and slightly to my

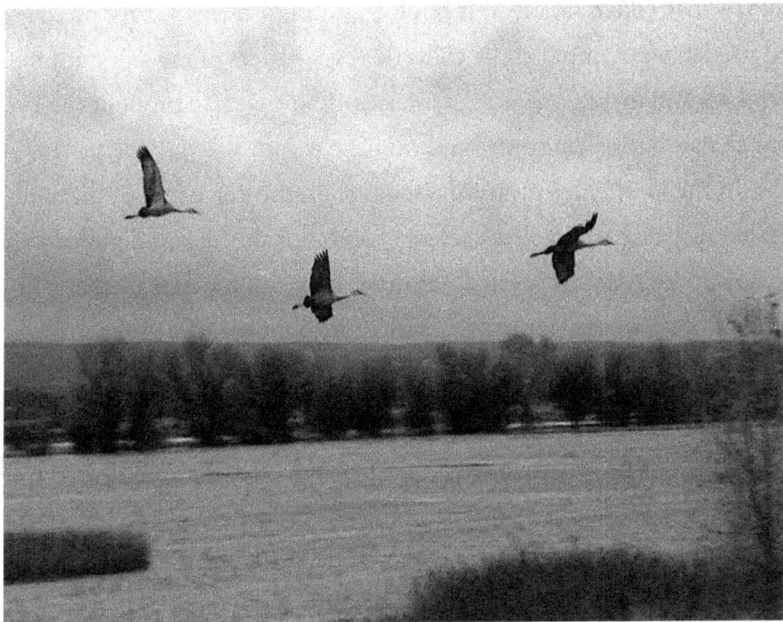

Sandhill cranes in the twilight at Bosque Del Apache National Wildlife Refuge

left, she delivered her comments with a dry sense of humor and a smile that lit up her face.

Some years into my tenure at the Y, I learned that Phoebe's beloved partner Nancy had experienced a relapse of the cancer that had been diagnosed five years earlier. Around that time, Phoebe had begun attending my t'ai chi ch'üan classes. Nancy's cancer went into remission for a while, but unfortunately its comeback was strong. During the next several months, the Schlessman YMCA t'ai chi ch'uan community – and the practice itself – seemed to be a gentle, steadying, and supportive element for Phoebe.

A while after Nancy's death, Phoebe and I talked about a trip she'd recently taken with family and friends, to the annual sandhill crane migratory stopover on the Platte River. During that visit, she told her family that, after her passing, she would like for her loved ones to scatter her and Nancy's ashes at that site in western Nebraska. Together, she said, they would ride the crane to the seven stars.

In that conversation, this book was born. Phoebe's story present-ed itself as an example of the collective experiences of my students, my teachers and myself...lived experiences of how we had brought the t'ai chi ch'üan out of the studio and into the world.

In the Grand Terminus, the focus is on the departure of the soul. It's no easy task to get to the release point, but the idea of flight carries a taste of joy. An unexpected lightness, long in preparation, like a lit-tle sigh. Just an easy letting go, with anticipation and without regret.

Joy Takes Wing

Performing the many t'ai chi ch'üan movements named for birds can help connect us to this state of being. As we contemplate the name and meaning while performing the sequences, we invite a cer-tain buoyancy of body, mind, and spirit. This can be discerned in ear-ly movements like Grasping the Bird's Tail, and later ones like Riding the Crane to the Seven Stars.

My mother often wore a silver necklace in the form of a crane tak-ing flight, and its simple shape brought a fond memory. About ten years before her death, she and I were strolling on the Highline Canal Trail in southeast Denver, a favorite spot just behind her apartment building. Off to the southeast, we spotted a group of about a half-doz-en big white birds, wheeling high in the blue sky. We concluded that they were whooping cranes.

My mother was a lifetime bird watcher. Like many others pursuing that pastime, she had a wish list of bird species she especially longed to see. After glimpsing those majestic birds, vivid white against a back-ground of blue, we rushed back to her apartment, flipped through the pages of *Peterson's Guide to Western Birds*, and pounced on the description of the whooping crane. Implausible as it seemed, we were convinced.

From that day on, we celebrated Crane Day every May 4. I bought her the crane necklace for Christmas that year, in honor of her con-nection to birds and in memory of that exciting day. It was a fleeting moment long ago, but the joy of it remains fresh.

I later deduced that the birds we saw were not whooping cranes, but pelicans. Maybe my mother knew that too, but it didn't matter to either of us. Pelicans are also white, also beautiful in flight, and often seen tracing graceful circles high in the air as they patrol for fish above bodies of water on Colorado's front range.

The Send-off of the Soul

Soon after we Ride the Crane to the Seven Stars, we move along in the current to another rich and compelling sequence: Shoot Out the Arrow. This is the final letting go. The left arm extends, the hand gently opens, and the soul departs.

In the t'ai chi ch'üan, as in our lives, we let go again and again. Finally, as we Shoot Out the Arrow, we arrive at the end of life. Then, all of our being must focus in on that one point – the opening of the hand and the gentle release of the soul.

Perhaps that opening hand can also contain the lotus flower that we just picked up…a taste of all that was beautiful and precious.

With that idea in mind, a few years ago I gathered with a group of the YMCA t'ai chi ch'üan students for one of our occasional outside practices. Catherine, a long-standing member of the group, had passed away peacefully in her sleep a few weeks before, and it felt right to give her a send-off. It was lilac blooming season, and I picked a few blossoms from the tree in my yard and brought them to the gathering. We shared them around, each person taking one or two of the individual flowers.

As always, we did the sequence in a green, shady corner of the park, facing a beautiful hawthorn tree whose branches had a sturdy, graceful growth habit. The sun came out and dappled its leaves and bark. After we performed Shoot Out the Arrow, we gently opened our hands and breathed out to give the flowers on our palms a little boost. As I drove home, the fragrance of other blooming lilac trees whispered to me through the open car window.

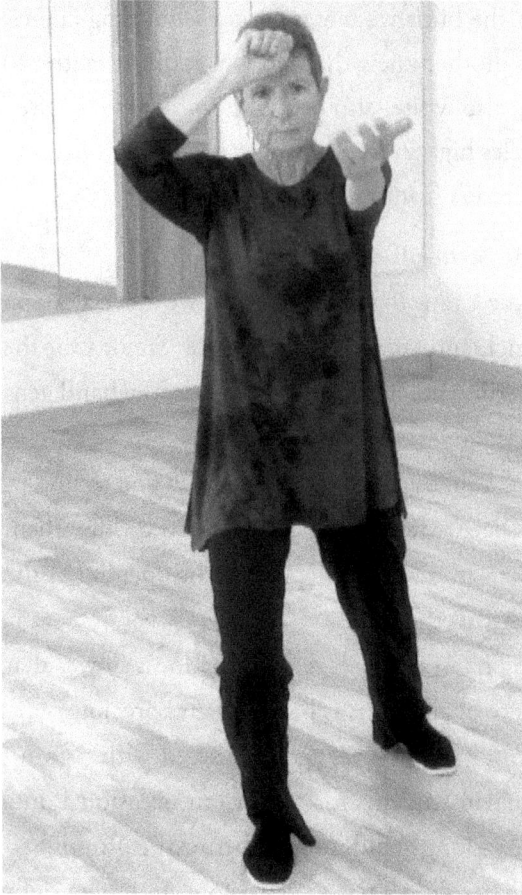

*After we shoot out
the arrow,
the hand opens
and the soul
takes flight.*

Since that spring day in 2019, I imagine at least 1,000 t'ai chi ch'üan "arrows" have been launched from that same shady spot. Less than a year after Catherine's death, the COVID-19 pandemic rewrote the script for the YMCA class, but later that year, a small group of former students began gathering in the park every week. I have no doubt that, had she lived, Catherine would have been among them, shooting out the arrow on Tuesday mornings toward the branches of the hawthorn tree.

In this sequence, we carefully focus the gaze on the gently opening hand – a very short moment arising from a very long preparation. In the epilogue of the second edition of *Looking for The Golden Needle,*

Gerda Geddes reflects on growing older, clearer, and lighter ahead of the transformation to come.

> So we rise from the vapours of the water and return to the water. This journey slowly reveals itself and the interpretation of the symbols slowly becomes more evident…The Snake Creeps Down Into the Water is the last major transformation, emptying us of everything, allowing us to float up Reaching for the Seven Stars.[8]

As for the upward and outward direction of the released soul from the outstretched hand, I offer one more lived experience. In September 2010, I stood knee-deep in the surf off of Cape Cod, facing east into the empty, pearly-grey Atlantic. In my hand was a shell containing a teaspoon-sized amount of my mother's ashes. Her body's journey ended here. I stretched out my hand, and an incoming wave caught up the shell and its contents with a joyful swoosh and an upward flourish. Later, I connected that moment to Gerda Geddes's words in the epilogue.

> The final stage, the Shooting Out of the Arrow, is a mystery. Where does the arrow go? We don't know. We just grow wider and deeper all the time and all we have to do is to climb to the top of the mountain and jump.[9]

Reflections of Mind, Body, and Intent

Phrases asking us to be "in the moment" can veer toward the trite and ambiguous, but the t'ai chi ch'üan offers us that opportunity. The Grand Terminus is an extra-special invitation. It's what we've been practicing for all along – being in the moment of transformation with grace and clarity. To ride the crane through the night skies to the seven stars and to witness the soul floating off into the ether invites us to be buoyant, nimble, and joyfully attentive. Then, we discover that the end is the beginning…a return to where we started.

Ride the crane, ride the tiger, shoot out the arrow. The names evoke a dramatic finish to the allegorical life journey. There is drama, energy, and physical challenge in the tightly scripted turns and weight shifts. All this is supported with love by the ground beneath the feet. When the torso follows the feet and the encircling arms, the whole body creates a spiraling energy that is rooted, supple, and centered.

At the end of this sequence, the fisted hand turns, then gently opens in the symbolic release of the soul. As we have just picked up the lotus flower, the symbol of life's fleeting beauty, the idea of release carries even more meaning. Throughout the form, fists contain energy; gently and securely held, not clenched or tight. Then the closed fist can open with power, focus, and grace, just as it did in Spoke of the Wheel and Twisting the Tiger's Ears. We've practiced and refined the art of letting go, just for this moment. Fisted hand, contained force, grounded energy, all released with clear intent, gratitude, and love.

Chapter Notes

Chapter 1

1. Dr. Yang, Jwing-Ming, *Tai Chi Chuan Classical Yang Style: The Complete Long Form and Qigong* (Wolfeboro, NH: YMAA Publication Center, 1999), 194.
2. Gerda Geddes, *Looking for The Golden Needle: An allegorical journey* (Plymouth PL3 4SX, Great Britain: MannaMedia, an imprint of Mannamead Press, 1991), 55.
3. "Bosque del Apache National Wildlife Refuge," U.S. Fish and Wildlife Service, accessed February 15, 2024, https://www.fws.gov/refuge/bosque-del-apache/about-us.
4. Benjamin Pang Jeng Lo, Martin Inn, Robert Amacker, and Susan Foe, eds. and trans., *The Essence of T'ai Chi Ch'uan*, (Berkeley, CA: Blue Snake Books, an imprint of North Atlantic Books, 1979), 88.

Chapter 2

1. Gerda Geddes, *Looking for The Golden Needle: An allegorical journey* (Plymouth PL3 4SX, Great Britain: Mannamead Press, 1991), 56.
2. Merriam-Webster.com, accessed February 15, 2024, https://www.merriam-webster.com/dictionary/chi
3. Yang Chengfu, *The Essence and Applications of Taijiquan*, trans. Louis Swaim (Berkeley, CA: Blue Snake Books, an imprint of North Atlantic Books, 2005), 117.
4. Yang Chengfu, *Taijiquan*, 27.
5. Yang Family Tai Chi Discussion Board, Yang Family Tai Chi, accessed January 19, 2023, https://discuss.yangfamilytaichi.com/viewtopic.php?t=1324
6. Poets.org, The Lake Isle of Innisfree, accessed March 25, 2024, https://poets.org/poem/lake-isle-innisfree

Chapter 3

1. Catalyst, Taijitu – What It Teaches Us About Ourselves, accessed January 26, 2023, https://catalystinspired.com/taijitu-symbol-yin-yang/
2. Jou, Tsung Hwa, *The Dao of Taijiquan: Way to Rejuvenation* (Scottsdale, AZ, Tai Chi Foundation, 2001), 111.
3. Bill Douglas and Angela Wong Douglas, *The Complete Idiot's Guide to T'ai Chi & Qi Gong* (New York, NY: Alpha Books, published by Penguin Group, 2020), 28.
4. Cheng Man-ch'ing, *Master Cheng's Thirteen Chapters On T'ai Chi Ch'üan,* Douglas Wile, translator (Brooklyn, NY, Sweet Ch'i Press, 1982), 76.
5. Gerda Geddes, *Looking for The Golden Needle: An allegorical journey* (Plymouth PL3 4SX, Great Britain: Mannamead Press, 1991), 57.
6. Yang Chengfu, *The Essence and Applications of Taijiquan,* Louis Swaim, translator (Berkeley, CA: Blue Snake Books, an imprint of North Atlantic Books, 2005), 31-32.
7. Geddes, *Looking for The Golden Needle*, 86.

Chapter 4

1. Dr. Yang, Jwing-Ming, *Tai Chi Chuan Classical Yang Style: The Complete Long Form and Qigong* (Wolfeboro, NH: YMAA Publication Center, 1999), 227.
2. Yang Chengfu, *The Essence and Applications of Taijiquan,* trans. Louis Swaim (Berkeley, CA: Blue Snake Books, an imprint of North Atlantic Books, 2005), 44-45.
3. Gerda Geddes, *Looking for The Golden Needle: An allegorical journey* (Plymouth PL3 4SX, Great Britain: Mannamead Press, 1991), 57-58.
4. Benjamin Pang Jeng Lo, Martin Inn, Robert Amacker, and Susan Foe, eds. and trans., *The Essence of T'ai Chi Ch'uan,* (Berkeley, CA: Blue Snake Books, an imprint of North Atlantic Books, 1979), 69.

5. Geddes, *Looking for The Golden Needle*, 58.
6. Lo, Inn, Amacker, and Foe, eds. and trans., *Essence of T'ai Chi Ch'uan*, 56.
7. Dr. Yang, Jwing-Ming, T*ai Chi Chuan Classical Yang Style*, 227.
8. Lo, Inn, Amacker, and Foe, eds. and trans., *Essence of T'ai Chi Ch'uan*, 69.

Chapter 5

1. Jou, Tsung Hwa, *The Dao of Taijiquan: Way to Rejuvenation* (Scottsdale, AZ: Tai Chi Foundation, 2001), 196.
2. Dr. Yang, Jwing-Ming, *Tai Chi Chuan Classical Yang Style: The Complete Long Form and Qigong* (Wolfeboro, NH: YMAA Publication Center, 1999), 235.
3. Gerda Geddes, *Looking for The Golden Needle: An allegorical journey* (Plymouth PL3 4SX, Great Britain: Mannamead Press, 1991), 58.
4. Jou, Tsung Hwa, *Dao of Taijiquan*, 23.

Chapter 6

1. Gerda Geddes, *Looking for The Golden Needle: An allegorical journey* (Plymouth PL3 4SX, Great Britain: Mannamead Press, 1991), 59.
2. Peter Wayne, with Mark L. Fuerst, *The Harvard Medical School Guide to Tai Chi* (Boulder, CO: Shambhala Publications, 2013), 111.
3. Wayne, *Harvard Medical School Guide to Tai Chi*, 119.
4. Yang Chengfu, *The Essence and Applications of Taijiquan*, trans. Louis Swaim (Berkeley, CA: Blue Snake Books, an imprint of North Atlantic Books, 2005), 11.
5. Geddes, *Looking for The Golden Needle*, 29.

6.   Bryan Robinson, Why You Hate Uncertainty, and How to Cope, Psychology Today, November 6, 2020, https://www.psychologytoday.com/us/blog/the-right-mindset/202011/why-you-hate-uncertainty-and-how-cope

Chapter 7

1.   Dr. Yang, Jwing-Ming, *Tai Chi Chuan Classical Yang Style: The Complete Long Form and Qigong* (Wolfeboro, NH: YMAA Publication Center, 1999), 243.
2.   Dr. Yang, Jwing-Ming, *Tai Chi Chuan Classical Yang Style,* 243.
3.   Peter Wayne, with Mark L. Fuerst, *The Harvard Medical School Guide to Tai Chi* (Boulder, CO: Shambhala Publications, 2013), 50-51.
4.   Yang Chengfu, *The Essence and Applications of Taijiquan,* trans. Louis Swaim (Berkeley, CA: Blue Snake Books, an imprint of North Atlantic Books, 2005), 115-116.
5.   Wayne, *The Harvard Medical School Guide to Tai Chi,* 91.
6.   Wayne, *The Harvard Medical School Guide to Tai Chi,* 91.
7.   Larry Cammarata, Eight Tai Chi Teaching Guidelines for Creating a Successful and Enjoyable Classroom Experience for New Students, accessed February 16, 2023, https://slantedflying.com/eight-tai-chi-teaching-guidelines-for-creating-a-successful-and-enjoyable-classroom-experience-for-new-students/
8.   Jill Bolte Taylor, *My Stroke of Insight: A Brain Scientist's Personal Journey* (New York, NY: Plume, a member of Penguin Group, 2009), 148.
9.   Gerda Geddes, *Looking for The Golden Needle: An allegorical journey* (Plymouth PL3 4SX, Great Britain: Mannamead Press, 1991), 60.

Chapter 8

1. Gerda Geddes, *Looking for The Golden Needle: An allegorical journey* (Plymouth PL3 4SX, Great Britain: Mannamead Press, 1991), 50-51.
2. Yang Chengfu, *The Essence and Applications of Taijiquan*, trans. Louis Swaim (Berkeley, CA: Blue Snake Books, an imprint of North Atlantic Books, 2005), 68-69.
3. Geddes, *Looking for The Golden Needle*, 60.
4. Geddes, *Looking for The Golden Needle*, 85.
5. Geddes, *Looking for The Golden Needle*, 91.
6. Geddes, *Looking for The Golden Needle*, 60.

Chapter 9

1. An Introduction to Buddhism Through Jodo Shinsu, accessed March 17, 2023, https://dharmanet.org/coursesM/Shin/JodoShinshu1a.htm
2. Gerda Geddes, *Looking for The Golden Needle: An allegorical journey* (Plymouth PL3 4SX, Great Britain: Mannamead Press, 1991), 60-61.
3. Jou, Tsung Hwa, *The Dao of Taijiquan: Way to Rejuvenation* (Scottsdale, AZ: Tai Chi Foundation, 2001), 196.
4. Dr. Yang, Jwing-Ming, *Tai Chi Chuan Classical Yang Style: The Complete Long Form and Qigong* (Wolfeboro, NH: YMAA Publication Center, 1999), 276.
5. Natural and Artificial Gaits of the Horse, accessed January 19, 2024, https://www.myhorseuniversity.com/single-post/2017/09/25/natural-and-artificial-gaits-of-the-horse
6. Geddes, *Looking for The Golden Needle*, 27.
7. Geddes, *Looking for The Golden Needle*, 30.

Chapter 10

1. Guanyin, accessed March 9, 2023, https://en.wikipedia.org/wiki/Guanyin

2. Christina Feldman, She Who Hears the Cries of the World, accessed March 31, 2023, https://www.lionsroar.com/she-who-hears-the-cries-of-the-world/

3. Gerda Geddes, *Looking for The Golden Needle: An allegorical journey* (Plymouth PL3 4SX, Great Britain: Mannamead Press, 1991), 61.

4. Dr. Yang, Jwing-Ming, *Tai Chi Chuan Classical Yang Style: The Complete Long Form and Qigong* (Wolfeboro, NH: YMAA Publication Center, 1999), 285.

5. Dr. Yang, Jwing-Ming, *Tai Chi Chuan Classical Yang Style*, 285.

6. Yang Chengfu, *The Essence and Applications of Taijiquan*, trans. Louis Swaim (Berkeley, CA: Blue Snake Books, an imprint of North Atlantic Books, 2005), 76.

7. Anne-Laure Le Cunff, "The Uncertain Mind: How the Brain Handles the Unknown," accessed February 16, 2024, https://nesslabs.com/uncertain-mind

8. "The Spirit Behind Aloha," accessed February 16, 2024, https://www.robertshawaii.com/blog/spirit-behind-aloha

9. Gerda Geddes, 1984, "TURNING POINTS." Unpublished article.

Chapter 11

1. Gerda Geddes, *Looking for The Golden Needle: An allegorical journey* (Plymouth PL3 4SX, Great Britain: Mannamead Press, 1991), 64.

2. Dr. Yang, Jwing-Ming, *Tai Chi Chuan Classical Yang Style: The Complete Long Form and Qigong* (Wolfeboro, NH: YMAA Publication Center, 1999), 298.

3. Dr. Yang, Jwing-Ming, *Tai Chi Chuan Classical Yang Style*, 299.

4. Jou, Tsung Hwa, *The Dao of Taijiquan: Way To Rejuvenation* (Scottsdale, AZ, Tai Chi Foundation, 2001), 166.
5. Waysun Liao, trans., *T'ai Chi Classics* (Boston, MA: Shambhala Publications, 1990), 117.
6. Jou, Tsung Hwa, *Dao of Taijiquan,* 198.
7. Jou, Tsung Hwa, *Dao of Taijiquan*, 198.
8. Geddes, *Looking for The Golden Needle,* 64.
9. Ed Berg, unpublished presentation, January 6, 2006.
10. Berg, unpublished presentation, January 6, 2006.
11. Berg, unpublished presentation, January 6, 2006.
12. Obituary of Edgar Lowndes Berg, Salida (CO) Mountain Mail (Salida, CO), October 17, 2022, https://www.themountainmail.com/obituaries/article_39dc7604-541d-11ed-a3f1-dbbcf1d99178.html.
13. Emily Dickinson, "A narrow Fellow in the Grass (1096)," accessed April 27, 2023, https://www.poetryoutloud.org/poem/a-narrow-fellow-in-the-grass-1096/
14. Rudyard Kipling, *The Jungle Book*, accessed April 27, 2023, https://www.telelib.com/authors/K/KiplingRudyard/prose/JungleBook/kaahunting.html

Chapter 12

1. Yang Chengfu, *The Essence and Applications of Taijiquan,* trans. Louis Swaim (Berkeley, CA: Blue Snake Books, an imprint of North Atlantic Books, 2005), 56.
2. Dr. Yang, Jwing-Ming, *Tai Chi Chuan Classical Yang Style: The Complete Long Form and Qigong* (Wolfeboro, NH: YMAA Publication Center, 1999), 248.
3. Gerda Geddes, *Looking for The Golden Needle: An allegorical journey* (Plymouth PL3 4SX, Great Britain: Mannamead Press, 1991), 121.
4. Cheng, Man-ch'ing, *Master Cheng's Thirteen Chapters On T'ai Chi Ch'üan*, trans. Douglas Wile (Brooklyn, NY: Sweet Ch'i Press, 1982), 73.

5. Benjamin Pang Jeng Lo, Martin Inn, Robert Amacker, and Susan Foe, eds. and trans., *The Essence of T'ai Chi Ch'uan,* (Berkeley, CA: Blue Snake Books, an imprint of North Atlantic Books, 1979), 85.

6. Lo, Inn, Amacker, and Foe, eds. and trans., *Essence of T'ai Chi Ch'uan,* 86.

7. Stephen T. Asma, "Was Bo Diddley a Buddha?," *New York Times,* April 10, 2017.

Chapter 13

1. Dr. Yang, Jwing-Ming, *Tai Chi Chuan Classical Yang Style: The Complete Long Form and Qigong* (Wolfeboro, NH: YMAA Publication Center, 1999), 328.

2. Dr. Yang, Jwing-Ming, *Tai Chi Chuan Classical Yang Style,* 328.

3. Dr. Yang, Jwing-Ming, *Tai Chi Chuan Classical Yang Style,* 329.

4. Dr. Yang, Jwing-Ming, *Tai Chi Chuan Classical Yang Style,* 329.

5. Dr. Yang, Jwing-Ming, *Tai Chi Chuan Classical Yang Style,* 329.

6. Dr. Yang, Jwing-Ming, *Tai Chi Chuan Classical Yang Style,* 330.

7. Gerda Geddes, Looking for *The Golden Needle: An allegorical journey* (Plymouth PL3 4SX, Great Britain: Mannamead Press, 1991), 65.

8. Geddes, *Looking for The Golden Needle,* 120-121.

9. Geddes, *Looking for The Golden Needle,* 125.

Selected Bibliography

Asma, Stephen T. "Was Bo Diddley a Buddha?" *New York Times,* April 10, 2017.

Berg, Edgar. Unpublished presentation, January 6, 2006. Private collection.

Bolte Taylor, Jill. *My Stroke of Insight: A Brain Scientist's Personal Journey.* New York: Plume, a member of Penguin Group, 2009.

Cammarata, Larry. "Eight Tai Chi Teaching Guidelines for Creating a Successful and Enjoyable Classroom Experience for New Students." Slanted Flying. September 3, 2018. https://slantedflying.com/eight-tai-chi-teaching-guidelines-for-creating-a-successful-and-enjoyable-classroom-experience-for-new-students.

Catalyst. "Taijitu—What It Teaches Us About Ourselves." Accessed March 19, 2024. https://catalystinspired.com/taijitu-symbol-yin-yang.

Cheng Man-ch'ing. *Master Cheng's Thirteen Chapters On T'ai Chi Ch'üan.* Douglas Wile, translator. Brooklyn: Sweet Ch'i Press, 1982.

Dharmanet. "An Introduction to Buddhism Through Jodo Shinsu." Accessed March 17, 2023. https://dharmanet.org/coursesM/Shin/JodoShinshu1a.htm.

Dickinson, Emily. "A narrow Fellow in the Grass (1096)." Poetry Out Loud. Accessed March 19, 2024. https://www.poetryoutloud.org/poem/a-narrow-fellow-in-the-grass-1096.

Douglas, Bill and Angela Wong. *The Complete Idiot's Guide to T'ai Chi & Qi Gong.* New York: Alpha Books, published by Penguin Group, 2020.

Feldman, Christina. "She Who Hears the Cries of the World." *Lion's Roar*. April 27, 2022. https://www.lionsroar.com/she-who-hears-the-cries-of-the-world.

Geddes, Gerda. *Looking for The Golden Needle: An allegorical journey*. Plymouth: MannaMedia, an imprint of Mannamead Press, 1991.

Jou Tsung Hwa. *The Dao of Taijiquan: Way to Rejuvenation*. Scottsdale: Tai Chi Foundation, 2001.

Kipling, Rudyard. *The Jungle Book*. Telelib. Accessed 2023. https://www.telelib.com/authors/K/KiplingRudyard/prose/Jungle-Book/kaahunting.html.

Le Cunff, Anne-Laure. "The Uncertain Mind: How the Brain Handles the Unknown." Ness Labs. Accessed February 16, 2024. https://nesslabs.com/author/annelaure.

Liao Waysun, translator. *T'ai Chi Classics*. Boston: Shambhala Publications, 1990.

Lo, Benjamin Pang Jeng; Inn, Martin; Amacker, Robert; and Foe, Susan, editors and translators. *The Essence of T'ai Chi Ch'uan*. Berkeley: Blue Snake Books, an imprint of North Atlantic Books, 1979.

Merriam-Webster. "Merriam-Webster Dictionary." Accessed March 28, 2024. https://www.merriam-webster.com/dictionary/chi

Mountain Mail (Salida, CO). Obituary of Edgar Lowndes Berg. October 17, 2022. https://www.themountainmail.com/obituaries/article_39dc7604-541d-11ed-a3f1-dbbcf1d99178.html.

My Horse University. "Natural and Artificial Gaits of the Horse." Accessed January 19, 2024. https://www.myhorseuniversity.com/single-post/2017/09/25/natural-and-artificial-gaits-of-the-horse.

Roberts Hawaii. "The Spirit Behind 'Aloha.'" Accessed March 19, 2024. https://www.robertshawaii.com/blog/spirit-behind-aloha/

Robinson, Bryan, "Why You Hate Uncertainty, and How to Cope."
    Psychology Today. November 6, 2020.
    https://www.psychologytoday.com/us/blog/the-right-
    mindset/202011/why-you-hate-uncertainty-and-how-cope.
U.S. Fish and Wildlife Service. "Bosque del Apache National
    Wildlife Refuge." Accessed February 15, 2024. https://www.
    fws.gov/refuge/bosque-del-apache/about-us.
Wayne, Peter, with Fuerst, Mark L. *The Harvard Medical School
    Guide to Tai Chi*. Boulder: Shambhala Publications, 2013.
Wikipedia. "Guanyin." Accessed March 19, 2024. https://en.wikipedia.
    org/wiki/Guanyin.
Yang Chengfu. *The Essence and Applications of Taijiquan*,
    Louis Swaim, translator. Berkeley: Blue Snake Books, an
    imprint of North Atlantic Books, 2005.
Yang Family Tai Chi. "Yang Family Tai Chi Discussion Board."
    Accessed January 19, 2024. https://discuss.yangfamilytaichi.
    com/viewtopic.php?t=1324.
Yang Jwing-Ming. *Tai Chi Chuan Classical Yang Style: The Complete
    Long Form and Qigong*. Wolfeboro: YMAA Publication
    Center, 1999.

www.ingramcontent.com/pod-product-compliance
Lightning Source LLC
Chambersburg PA
CBHW060902280326
41934CB00007B/1155